VAGUS NERVE:

THE GUIDE TO HEAL DEPRESSION AND ANXIETY BY FINDING BALANCE IN YOUR LIFESTYLE.

STIMULATE THE VAGUS NERVE TO PREVENT THE NERVE'S INFLAMMATION TO IMPROVE YOUR BODY AND MENTAL HEALTH.

By Practicing Mindfulness

© Copyright 2020 Practicing Mindfulness – All rights reserved.

The content contained within this book may not be reproduced, duplicated or transmitted without direct written permission from the author or the publisher.

Under no circumstances will any blame or legal responsibility be held against the publisher, or author, for any damages, reparation, or monetary loss due the information contained within this book. Either directly or indirectly.

Legal Notice:

This book is copyright protected. This book is only for personal use. You cannot amend, distribute, sell, use, quote or paraphrase any part, or the content within this book, without the consent of the author or the publisher.

Disclaimer Notice:

Please note the information contained within this document is for educational and entertainment purposes only. All effort has been executed to present accurate, up to date, and reliable, complete information. No warranties of any kind are declared or implied. Readers acknowledge that the author is not engaging in the rendering of legal, financial, medical or professional advice. The content of this book has been derived from many sources. Please consult a licensed professional before attempting any technique outlined in this book.

By reading this document, the reader agrees that under no circumstances is the author responsible of any losses, direct or indirect, which are incurred as a result of the use of the information contained within this document, including, but not limited to, - errors, omissions, or inaccuracies.

Table Of Contents

Introduction 1

What Is The Vagus Nerve And Where Is Located? 4

The Functions Of Vagus Nerve 18

What Is Depression? 32

Signs Of Depression 38

What Is Anxiety? 42

Signs Of Anxiety 54

The Relation Between Vagus Nerve And Depression ... 66

Symptoms Of Vagus Nerve Inflammation 79

What Happens If The Vagus Nerve Is Damaged? 94

How To Stimulate Vagus Nerve 113

Activating Your Vagus Nerve Effortlessly 122

Why Is Important To Organise A Good Routine And Don't Ignore Hobbies And Passions 132

Few Tips To Have A Good Routine 143

Conclusion 156

Introduction

On a daily basis, we run through one emotion to the next, from happy to sad to angry to afraid, often without giving any question or attention to them for longer than a few minutes. But, with the increase of mental health disorders on the rise, you may question whether our bodies are actually designed to handle the high stress or traumatic events so many have struggled to overcome?

What can be more alarming is the additional health problems that arise from what are typically considered mood or emotional disorders. Individuals are at greater risk of heart disease, respiratory infection, and digestive complications when they struggle with cognitive and/or mental issues. While many types of therapies address the thoughts and feelings that cause emotional stress and medication help manage symptoms of the physical health condition, what seems to be overlooked is what actually connects mental disorders with physical complications?

The body is filled with complex systems that regulate movement, sensory information, organ function, and hormone production. These systems often directly or indirectly connect and have an impact on one another.

The brain, heart, lungs, and digestive system, for instance, are all connected by one nerve. It is the heart of the brain-body connection. It is this nerve that can be the common link between mental health disorders and other physical health conditions.

Individuals who suffer from depression, autism spectrum disorder, chronic illnesses, and trauma struggle on a daily basis to find relief from their symptoms. While therapy can provide them with coping mechanisms, they still often have difficulty maintaining a healthy and peaceful state of mind. This book is designed to help those individuals who struggle with some of these common disorders. It can also provide valuable information to those who want to prevent and avoid these conditions and other physical health problems.

In this book, you will learn the inner workings of the body's complex autonomic nervous system. This system is responsible for regulating mood, emotions, heart rate, digestion, speech, hearing, and more. It is in this system you learn about the vagus nerve; the nerve that links the brain with the rest of the body and directly impacts how stress and emotions affect the proper function of vital organs.

You will find specific exercises, activities, and tips that can help you strengthen this nerve to combat depression, anxiety, PTSD, chronic illness, among others. While it is designed to provide hope, relief, and answers to those who suffer from mental or health disorder, it is a book that can positively impact all who read it. What you are about to learn is that our bodies have evolved to properly deal with any stress and/or emotions it newly encounters.

What Is The Vagus Nerve And Where Is Located?

For your body to function properly, it relies on a system of nerves. A nerve simply refers to a whitish fiber that transmits impulses in your body from the brain to the spinal cord and to the muscles. Although there are different types of nerves, the primary role played by all nerves is to transmit sensory impulses between the brain and the rest of the body. Without nerves, communication between the brain and the other parts of the body would be impossible. The brain cannot send signals to the rest of the body if the nerves fail to function. The combination of all the nerves in the body forms the autonomic nervous system.

The nervous system is a very complex part of the body that that ensures that the functions of each nerve are coordinated and that sensory signals are transmitted throughout the body. Think of the nervous system as a production and supply coordination process. In a production company, there are many workers working on different levels to attain the same purpose. This is the same concept that is applied in the functioning of the nervous system. The system is well coordinated to ensure that the independent roles played by each nerve lead to the well-functioning of the body. At the end of the day, each independent action taken by the body must lead to the proper functioning of the entire body.

The nervous system is so complex that it can detect environmental changes instantly. If you did not have nerves, the body would not be able to detect temperature changes. People who suffer damaged nerves suffer from a lack of senses. A person may even hold on to a hot pan and miss feeling the heat burning up their hand if the sensory nerves are damaged. This explains how important nerves are to all of us. The nervous system does not work independently. There is continuous coordination between the nervous system, the brain, and the endocrine system.

The endocrine system is a collection of glands that secrets hormones according to the signals being sent by the nervous system. Without the endocrine system, it is impossible for the body to respond to the signals being sent by the nervous system. For instance, when you eat, the nervous system communicates that a certain type of food has been introduced to the body. It is the signal from the nervous system that prompts the release of the necessary hormones for food digestion. This shows the importance of the nervous system in the overall running of your body. The system determines all the actions you take and dictates the functions of the body. The system controls blood flow and dictates what you do in different situations.

There are many endocrine glands in humans and other animals. In humans, the main endocrine glands are thyroid and adrenal glands. These two glands are responsible for releasing chemicals and hormones that affect our emotions and also control the digestive system. As we will observe later, all these factors are linked to the vagus nerve.

The Vagus Nerve is the longest and the most complex nerve in the nervous system. In reality, the vagus nerve comprises three parts, but they are commonly referred to as the vagus nerve. The nerve is part of the 12 cranial nerves, starting from the brain all the way to the spinal cord and other parts of the body. The nerve mainly transmits information from the surface of the brain tissue to the other parts of the body.

The term vagus is a Latin word, meaning wandering. The vagus nerve is very long as compared to the other cranial nerves, and it accesses most parts of the body. Due to its length and complexity, it is thought to be wandering and hence the name vagus.

The nerve, which is the tenth cranial nerve, was historically known as the pneumogastric nerve. It has an interface with the parasympathetic glands. They work together to control the heart, lungs, and digestive system. The nerve is the longest in the autonomic nervous system. The nerve ends at a very sensitive part known as the spinal accessory nucleus.

The two branches of sensory nerve cells of the vagus nerve serve as the central communication system between the brain and the body. This nerve offers multiple body functions that contribute largely to the nervous system. The nerve is known for the parasympathetic and sympathetic functions. It is primarily responsible for sensory and motor actions, as we will see later on too.

In simple terms, the vagus nerve is the link that connects the neck, heart, lungs, and the abdomen to the brain. These parts of the body are vital and very necessary for the well-being of any person. For this reason, the vagus nerve has been cited by many medical professionals as the center of human well-being. If your nerve is in good health and functioning properly, you are likely to function properly. However, any problems with the vagus nerve may lead to other problems in your health. Complications relating to your breathing, blood pressure, and your mental health are all linked to the vagus nerve.

Where Is the Nerve Located

The vagus nerve is known as the longest one because of its wide distribution. There is no specific location in the body where you can point out to be the location of the nerve. As a matter of fact, this nerve is distributed so widely that it touches all the important parts of the body. Like all other important cranial nerves, the vagus nerve starts from the brain.

The nerve runs from the brain through the neck and thorax and finally ends in the abdomen. The nerve has many branches and distributions along this route. The fact that that the nerve is made up of parasympathetic fibers and the fact that it is distributed in sensory glands makes its distribution even more complex. The vagus nerve has two main sensory ganglia. These are mainly the masses of tissue that transmit impulses. The ganglia are further divided into two, the superior and the inferior ganglia. The minor branches of the superior ganglion end up in the ear from the skin of the ear, ending up at the concha. The inferior ganglion, on the other hand, is further divided into two branches, the superior laryngeal nerve and the pharyngeal. The laryngeal breaks from the primary vagus at the lower neck but before the upper thorax. This nerve is very vital for speech coordination since it ends up at the larynx (The voice box). At this stage, the nerve also gives out the esophageal, cardiac, and pulmonary branches. Further lower, the vagus nerve extends to the digestive system.

Given that the nerve has the most widely distributed network, it makes sense that it plays an important role in human functioning. Although it is just part of the 12 cranial nerves, it has stood out to be one of the most reliable and critical anatomical features in the human body. Any interference or failure may be fatal. Its pharyngeal and laryngeal branches are responsible for motor impulses. The cardiac branch is primarily important in controlling the heartbeat while the esophageal branch acts in controlling your breathing. The bronchial branch acts to constrict bronchi muscles. These branches are vital in controlling involuntary muscles in the stomach, gallbladder, pancreas, and the small intestines.

Considering that the nerve is very central and that it links to most parts of the body, it is commonly used as a point of reference when checking the lifeline of a person. The vagus nerve stimulation done by applying an electric shock can be used to help patients who suffer from epilepsy, Alzheimer's, and migraines regain consciousness.

Why Is the Nerve Important

As we have seen, the vagus nerve is perhaps the most important of the 12 cranial nerves in the human body. But why exactly is the vagus nerve termed as being very important? Early studies on the nerve were misconstrued to suggest that the vagus was just like any other among the 12 cranial nerves. However, advancements in technology and a much more improved understanding of human anatomy have proved that the nerve is indeed the most important.

First, you must consider the fact that it covers a large part of the body, providing support for the most critical functions. Running from the head, through the neck, the thorax to the lower abdomen, the vagus nerve is definitely important to the functioning of the body.

The vagus is the body's primary parasympathetic nerve; hence, it supplies parasympathetic fibers throughout the upper body, including the head, neck, chest, and abdomen. This makes the central nerve in controlling your actions and motions even when you are sick. The nerve is responsible for the gag reflex. The nerve is also beneficial in that it helps control the heart rate, controlling sweating, regulation of blood pressure, and controlling vascular tone. Most people fail to understand the role played by the vagus nerve when it comes to balancing a fully functional body. If any of the above-mentioned physiological factors get out of hand, a person may suffer serious illnesses. Some of these aspects may lead to mental diseases, while others are responsible for instantaneous attacks such as cardiac arrest.

The Vasovagal Reflex: One of the most important benefits of the vagus nerve is the regulation of vasovagal reflex. When the nerve is stimulated suddenly, it leads to a physiological reaction known as vasovagal reflex. This state of the body entails a sudden drop in blood pressure and a slow heart rate. Most people often confuse this state of the body with heart attacks. Vasovagal reflection can be triggered by certain illnesses such as gastrointestinal conditions, or it can also be triggered by traumatic occurrences. In all instances, the vagus nerve must be controlled to help the victims. If these conditions lead to the sudden stimulation of the vagus nerve, and a person falls into a state of vasovagal reflex, it is just reasonable that the patient must be helped immediately. In some people, the reflex happens more often than in others. When a person undergoes vasovagal reflex, they are likely to lose their consciousness due to overthinking.

The vagus nerve is also important in that it plays a primary role in calming down patients. Excessive activation of the nerve has been proved to have a therapeutic effect on people suffering from Supraventricular tachycardia (SVT), an abnormally rapid heart rhythm. It has also been proven that the nerve can be used as a principal point of analysis. Many doctors use the nerve to diagnose many conditions, such as heart murmurs. The use of the Valsalva maneuver to stimulate the vagus nerve can be employed to help doctors carry out certain diagnoses.

The Vagus Nerve and the Heart: The vagus nerve also plays an important role in controlling the heartbeat and regulating blood flow. The right nerve supplies the sinus node. This means that any stimulation to the right vagus nerve can lead to the production of sinus bradycardia. On the other hand, the left vagus nerve supplies the AV node. This means that its stimulation may lead to the production of a heart block. Through the production of heart block, the Valsalva is in a position to undergo maneuver for the sake of terminating various kinds of SVT.

The Vagus Nerve in Medical Therapy: The study of the vagus nerve has revealed that it is one of the most outstanding organs of the body. Many scientists have been interested in using the nerve for therapeutic purposes. Currently, nerve stimulation and vagus nerve blocking are the main approaches that are employed when using the nerve in therapy.

For several years, a procedure known as vagotomy was employed to help treat patients suffering from stomach ulcers. It was realized that vagotomy (cutting of the vagus nerve) helped reduce the amount of peptic acid being produced. However, this application had several side effects and had to be abandoned. Still, efforts have been made by doctors to try and utilize the resources attached to the nerve for the sake of treatment. Although some doctors still use vagotomy, the practice has subsided due to other alternative treatment methods that are less harmful.

With that said, the vagus nerve is still a source of many treatments. Today, most medical practitioners are interested in chronic vagus nerve stimulation. This is a practice that has been found effective in treating various medical conditions, including severe epilepsy. Doctors use a vagus nerve stimulating device (VNS) to try and apply chronic stimulation to such patients. The same technique is used to treat patients who suffer from refractory depression.

The application of VNS devices has been overestimated. In recent years, many companies that manufacture VNS devices have advertised them as the ultimate solution to various conditions. Some are still carrying out tests on the use of VNS devices when it comes to the treatment of hypertension and tinnitus. While the fact that stimulating the vagus nerve positively affects your health is true, there are many lies propagated about the nerve. Before you spend your money on any otherwise medical process that is not recommended by a professional doctor, you should do proper research. Do not be in a hurry to dash out your money based on false advertisements or based on information that does not have medical support.

Thankfully, many institutions are now picking up the pace in researching about such products. In one study conducted by The Harvard Health School, it was found that VNS devices were effective in treating epilepsy. For the 21 individuals who were used in the study, 90% reported improvements health-wise during the first year. However, after 3 years, some patients started reporting relapse. This study was only based on VNS devices produced by one manufacturer. It is a long time since 2004, and many improvements have been made to the technology. With that said, it is still vital for any person seeking to undergo VNS to have the right information from the right sources. You must scrutinize every content you come across and try to compare facts by carrying out individual research.

The Biological Aspects That Make Vagus Nerve Important

It is a fact that the vagus nerve is the most important of all nerves in cranial order. However, some people fail to understand why. Here are some biological facts that can explain the extent to which this nerve may be of importance.

It Is Widespread: It is probably the most widespread nerve; starting from the brain to the thorax, and finally to the abdomen. In all sections of the body, the nerve is further subdivided into other small nerves. For instance, the esophageal and the cardiac and the pulmonary branches in the thorax conduct totally different purposes, that are pivotal to human survival. The esophageal primarily stimulates the esophagus and ensures the proper running of these areas of the body. On the other hand, pulmonary and cardiac extensions play a major role in controlling your blood flow and heart rate. You realize that all these factors are vital for human survival. If you do not enjoy a steady blood flow or continuous breathing, you are likely to die. The need of the vagus nerve to control such aspects cannot be underestimated. Any stimulation to nerve also affects such critical functions.

Links to Endocrine Glands: The fact that the vagus nerve links to important endocrine glands also shows that it is a vital part of your body. The endocrine glands play a major role in determining the functions or actions taken by your body. As we have mentioned above, the endocrine system coordinates with the nervous system to see that important chemicals and hormones are released in the body when necessary. This makes the vagus nerve a central part in the functioning of many bodily activities. The major endocrine glands include pineal glands, pituitary glands, ovaries, pancreas, thyroid, testes, parathyroid, and adrenal glands. All these glands are vital for the performance of day to day activities such as sexual intercourse, eating, breathing, sweating, among others. For instance, the adrenal glands are responsible for the production of adrenaline, which happens during moments of tension. This means that the vagus nerve can affect your adrenalin production and as a result, can affect your emotions and moods. The stimulation of your vagus nerve may also affect your emotions and even sexual desire. However, all these factors are subject to scientific proof. Although science has pointed out some direct relationships between the hormone secretion and the stimulation of the vagus nerve, it is not an outrightly black and white situation. Several anatomical factors count when it comes to the generation of hormones and starting any physiological process.

The Functions Of Vagus Nerve

The vagus nerve plays an important role in fulfilling bodily functions, as we have already observed. In this chapter, we will be looking at the details of each of the functions performed by the vagus nerve in association with the nervous system. It is important to note that the vagus nerve is a part of the autonomous nervous system and does not act as an independent entity. Some of the functions outlined in this chapter are achieved when the vagus nerve works in coordination with other cranial nerves. There are two primary roles of the vagus nerve, sympathetic and parasympathetic functions.

Sympathetic Functions

The sympathetic functions of the vagus nerve are thought to counteract the functions of the parasympathetic nerve. The main difference between the two is that the sympathetic functions occur in a conscious state while the parasympathetic functions occur in a subconscious state. This means that the parasympathetic functions of the vagus nerve are supposed to occur when the body is at rest. On the contrary, sympathetic functions encourage hyperactivity.

The sympathetic nervous system SNS is known for mediating the hormonal stress response and neuronal function. The nerve is central in starting a fight or flight response in the body. The flight or fight response refers to hormonal changes that occur when a person is nervous or in a dangerous situation. The common hormone that is excreted during this state is adrenaline. The fight or flight response is referred to as sympathoadrenal because it depends on the adrenal glands to generate high levels of adrenaline.

The entire process of response to threats, which may lead to fight or flight response is transmitted through the sympathetic nervous system, which is mainly supported by the vagus nerve. The transmission of impulses and hormonal action is supported by the nerve and enhanced by catecholamine secreted by the adrenal medulla. When this process happens, it directly affects the cardiac functions. For example, stimulation of the sympathetic nervous system can lead to the widening of bronchial passages, increased heart rate, constriction of blood vessels, and decreased motility of large intestines.

When the sympathetic nervous system is in action, the body is likely to experience increased or decreased temperature. Some theorists believe that the SNS was used in early organisms to support survival since most organisms had to be ready for action at any moment. It has been observed that sympathetic activity in humans increases moments before waking up, which prepares a person for daily activities. As an individual, you must find a way of stimulation your sympathetic nervous system. If you want to be active and productive in any area of your life, it is important to ensure that your body is active and positively ready to face all the challenges. The response of the sympathetic nervous system takes away feelings of laziness and fatigue. If your body is in an active state, you will feel energetic and active.

The Fight-Or-Flight Response

The other important function of the vagus nerve is the fight or flight response, which is essentially a part of the sympathetic nervous system. The use of the term fight or flight was first introduced by psychologist Walter Cannon. In his theory, he states that animals respond to threats by discharging their sympathetic nervous system, preparing the animal to either fight off the threat or retreat.

Catecholamine hormones are key in the process of preparation for fight or flight action. Such hormones include adrenaline and noradrenalin, which facilitates the immediate action of the muscles in preparation for a violent encounter.

There are obvious physiological and physical signs that outwardly show a person's state of emotion due to the activation of the hormones related to fighting or flight. Some of the conscious physiological reactions include:

• Increase heart rate or lung action, in which case, a person can be seen breathing heavily, or you may feel your heart skip a bit.

• Hot flashes or paling; in some instances, a person may experience both.

• Slowdown of digestion may occur in some individuals due to inhibiting of the stomach and upper intestinal action.

• Constriction of blood vessels in most parts of the body, which may affect the heart rate and blood pressure.

• Dilation of blood vessels may also occur in some individuals.

• Inhibiting the activities of lacrimal glands, which are responsible for salivation and tear production.

- Relaxation of the blood, which may result in the wetting of your clothes during a dangerous situation.

- Erection dysfunction during the moments of tension.

- Sometimes may result in loss of hearing

- May result in loss of peripheral vision, which means that the patient only has a smaller field of view.

In ancient times, the fight or flight response was manifested in a much different perspective from our modern world. In the early days, the fight response was associated with aggressive violent and combative behavior. In those days, the masculinity of a male person was measured upon the combative techniques. It was common for people to solve issues through combat. However, times have changed, and so has the aspects of fight and flight. Generally, the ancient world only associated the flight response with a predatory situation, where the victim did not have any other way out but to flee. This includes dangerous situations such as being attacked by a wild animal.

Today, the fight and flight response is manifested in many ways. For example, the fight response might be manifested through argumentative logical debates while the flight response may take several forms, including social withdrawal, silence, substance abuse, overeating, viewing television, among others. If you are not keen, you may fail to notice the parasympathetic action related to the fight or flight response in the modern world. Many people still expect people to use combative techniques used in ancient days. However, modern-day responses are very unique and need a keen eye for interpretation.

With that said, it is also important to note that males and females handle stress differently. Even in the early days, males were expected to react to stressful situations through an aggressive fight. On the other hand, it was expected of ladies to flee the situation. The same case applies in the modern world with a more open-minded perspective. Today, men are not expected to be heroes or fighters in all situations. It is okay for a man to flee a dangerous situation, and it is okay for a lady to stand and fight.

Parasympathetic Functions

The other important function of the vagus nerve is the parasympathetic function. As already mentioned, this function of the nerve tends to counteract the actions of the sympathetic nervous system. Although both parasympathetic and sympathetic actions of the vagus nerve work together, they are intended to perform contrary actions. This is one of the reasons why the vagus nerve must be considered as a part of the autonomous nervous system. Without having a regulatory mechanism in place, it would be virtually impossible for the nervous system to function appropriately. The system has to work in line with the vagus nerve and endocrine glands.

The parasympathetic nerves are important in stimulating several body functions among the sexual arousal, lacrimation, salivation, digestion, urination, and defecation. Most of these processes occur subconsciously; however, some have to take place consciously. Given that most processes occur subconsciously, it becomes difficult for most people to control these actions during sympathetic response situations. Parasympathetic processes that occur subconsciously, such as urination, may be adversely affected during sympathetic actions such as fight or flight response.

Parasympathetic Nervous System PSNS mainly uses acetylcholine as the primary transmitter. Other transmitters may be used where deemed necessary, e.g., the use of cholecystokinin peptides.

The Parasympathetic Nervous System

The parasympathetic nervous system is a part of the autonomic nervous system. This section of the nervous system also depends on the vagus nerve as the primary sensory nerve, among others. Just like the sympathetic nervous system, the parasympathetic system cannot operate in a vacuum. The vagus nerve functions in conjunction with other cranial nerves of the autonomic nerves system. The Autonomic nervous system ANS acts as the overall control system that coordinates the functions of all the nerves in the body. The actions of the parasympathetic nervous system would otherwise be in conflict with those of the sympathetic nervous system,

The ANS works to see that the nerves and various glands are controlled unconsciously. This means that the system gives signals for stimulating action among various nerves and glands. The ANS gives the go-ahead for actions to take place, which means that it is responsible for stimulation of rest and digestive activities such as salivation, sexual arousal, urination, defecation, and digestion.

The actions of the ANS are referred to as complementary to the actions of the other branches of the nervous system. In simpler terms, since the parasympathetic and the sympathetic nervous systems work in opposition to each other, there is a need to have regulatory measures. Due to the presence of the ANS, the parasympathetic and the sympathetic are viewed as complementary and not antagonistic as it would be without regulatory mechanisms.

We can consider the sympathetic nervous response as a quick response, which helps mobilize systems. On the other hand, the parasympathetic is a slow response system that is slowly activated but has a higher impact once in place.

As we have observed, the primary functions of the parasympathetic nervous system include salivation, urination, lacrimation, digestion, and defecation. The parasympathetic division depends to a large extent on the vagus nerve on performing such duties. We have seen that this division of the nervous system mainly relies on acetylcholine (ACh) neurotransmitters and sometimes may use peptides such as cholecystokinin. ACh acts on the muscarinic and nicotinic receptors. This primarily involves the stimulation of the vagus nerve, to release

ACh at the ganglion. It is the ACh, which then acts on nicotinic receptors, leading to the actions of the PSNS. As you can see, the stimulation of the vagus nerve is an integral part of the actions of the PSNS and that the activities of the nerve are vital for your survival. You can't underestimate the influence of the nerve that controls your digestion, urination, defecation, among other key bodily activities.

Sensory Functions

The vagus nerve, as a part of the nervous system, plays other roles that are not primary. In the sensory functions of the nerve, we come across the somatic functions (sensation from the skin and some muscles) and visceral functions. These functions facilitate the operations of the body in general. The auricular nerve, which innervates the skin along the external auditory part of the canal and external ear, is of great importance.

The important functions of the vagus nerve on the upper thorax include Laryngopharynx, which occurs within the laryngeal nerve. The more important aspects of the nerve are felt at the larynx, which includes the control and coordination of speech through the internal laryngeal nerve. The vagus nerve also functions as the central sensory nerve for the gastrointestinal tract through the terminal branches of the nerve. Observation of the heart through the cardiac branches reveals that the vagus nerve also plays a central role in determining the well-being of the heart, helping stimulate the heart muscles into pumping actions. The nerve also influences the contraction and dilation of arteries or veins that are close to the heart, having a great influence on the overall health of your heart.

With that in mind, this nerve has also been found to have a minor function in the detection of taste. Different fibers from the tongue and the epiglottis are linked to the nerve. However, this does not in any way mean that the vagus nerve is the primary sensory nerve when it comes to taste. The glossopharyngeal nerve caters to over 1/3 of the taste sensation on the tongue. However, the vagus nerve becomes very vital because it coordinates certain actions within the autonomic nervous system, which help kickstart the process of hormone generation for food digestion, among others.

Motor Functions

One of the most important actions of the vagus nerve is motor. When it comes to starting an activity within the muscle and prompting movements, the vagus nerve works to see that such actions take place subconsciously. For instance, the vagus nerve innervates the majority of the muscles, which are associated with the larynx and the pharynx. Such muscles are responsible for the initiation of critical muscular activities such as swallowing and phonation. Thanks to the active vagus activities, you can constantly swallow saliva without having to focus on it consciously.

Most muscles in the pharynx are linked to the pharyngeal branches of the vagus nerve. This should be seen as a positive aspect of the nerve since it plays a role in the coordination of the muscles in this area. Some of the actions initiated by the vagus include pharyngeal muscle constriction and palatopharyngeal.

The vagus nerve is also primary in coordinating the motor activities of the larynx. This is achieved through recurrent activities of the laryngeal nerve. As we have observed, the laryngeal nerve is one of the important branches of the vagus at the neck right before the thorax. This nerve functions by coordinating with other sensory glands such as thyroarytenoid and posterior Enrico-arytenoid.

Besides the pharynx and the larynx, the vagus nerve also has an effect on the palatoglossus and the soft palate parts of your tongue. These actions are important and are all indications of the superiority of the vagus nerve.

As we delve much deeper, we will be looking at other functions of the vagus nerve and their application to your daily life. In essence, we have mainly focused on the anatomical aspects of the nerve up to this stage. Before we move on to the next section, it is important to try and sum up the important points captured above.

- The vagus nerve is a nerve that runs from the brain through the neck, thorax, and lower abdomen. This nerve is the 10th of the 12 cranial nerves. It is a part of the autonomic nervous system and functions in coordination with the autonomic nervous system

- The vagus nerve is subdivided into several sections starting from the neck to the abdomen. Different branches of the nerve perform different functions. For instance, the laryngeal moves to the ears and is vital in controlling the sensory actions of the hearing and the vocal aspects of a person. The branches carry out different functions in relation to the nervous system.

- The functions of the vagus nerve are coordinated by the autonomic nervous system and are divided into sympathetic and parasympathetic. Although all these functions are sensory, they counter each other. While the sympathetic functions promote hyperactivity, the parasympathetic actions lead the body to a state of rest. The differences within the sensory actions of the nerve are dealt with by the ANS, which functions as a complementary component. However, it is also important to remember that the nervous system does not entirely depend on the vagus nerve as it has been made to sound in the public domain.

What Is Depression?

Depression is caused by changes in life circumstances, grief, stress, alterations in hormone levels, medical conditions, and several other traumatic and overwhelming demands of life. These factors alter the brain chemistry. The onset of depression and its expression differs among people. How people deal with grief is in part influenced by their genetic patterns.

Depression is linked to the state of our heart, our heart is linked to our emotions or feelings, and our emotions or feelings are linked to our thoughts. If you feel overwhelmed or anxious about a situation or unforeseen circumstances have made a significant impact in your life, and you don't get the right psychological support or tools to help you, this can have a long-term effect on the state of your heart and mental health. Deferred hope and storing anxiety in our heart can weigh us down, causing us to experience depression. This is why the mental illness approach to depression can keep us stuck in a cycle of depression because it doesn't give us hope that we will ever be able to move forward and live a life free from depression. We need to take a new approach when providing therapy to people who suffer from depression, and that approach is giving them the strategies to improve their mental health which provides them with hope instead of teaching people they will always have a mental illness.

Often, we focus solely on our minds when it comes to depression. Yes, our minds are essential but our heart, emotions, and thoughts are all interrelated, and we must pay attention to all of these precious parts of our inner self and physical body. I completely respect the medical field and all the fantastic people who work in that industry. However, the medical field often treats our physical symptoms and diagnoses our situations based on what our physical body is telling us, but how did we get to that state in the first place? When we seek help from a medical doctor, they are not extensively trained in the field of psychological development, and they don't have the time to listen to our most profound thoughts that lead to our emotional issues or the state of our heart. Expecting them to be able to fix depression when the cause isn't a physical issue, will continue to lead us down a road of defeat when it comes to depression.

The physical symptoms of depression are often said to be caused by a chemical imbalance in the brain and are treated with a drug based on this symptom. We can't merely take medication and expect our depression to be healed. The cause must be dealt with if we want our mental health to improve or change permanently. Medication might help to relieve some of the symptoms we are experiencing but we need to realize medication alone is not going to cure our depression. As a society, we have become lazy and accustomed to fast food convenience expecting all of our answers to be given to us in a prescription. Life can be hard, and sometimes we have to make changes that we might not necessarily want to make. However, if we are going to improve our mental health and live a life free of depression, we need to take action to make choices that are healthy for us as individuals.

If your job, living situation, environment or relationships are causing you to experience toxic emotions continually, you may have to decide to change the way you are reacting to those circumstances or leave that situation altogether. Our mental health is just as important as our physical health, and we need to be wise in determining what we allow to effect our emotions. If we take this approach to our mental health on a daily basis, this will protect us from experiencing long-term mental health issues.

When we begin to understand ourselves, we will naturally be drawn to the people who are like us, and we can learn to grow into the person we were created to be. We will begin to love ourselves, even when the people around us are not showing love towards us.

If you're unhappy, maybe you don't know who you are, and you are trying to fit into an environment that doesn't understand you? When we try to put a puzzle together, and we put a piece in the wrong place, it doesn't fit, right? We need the right parts in the right areas for the puzzle to be completed.

The Causes of depressions

The faulty mood causes this disorder. The emotion is about the general feeling one has about a specific event or a person. This aspect can also be called as an attitude or the public emotions people have. Moods can be positive or negative. Some positive moods include joy, happiness, a feeling of self-worthiness, and many others. However, when considering depression, it is associated with bad attitudes, which involves one being sad, anxious, low self-esteem, anger, narcissistic, arrogance, and many other emotions.

Other specialists believe this menace originates from the genes. They say that like 'father like son. Therefore, if the parent experiences some personality disorder, the offspring is likely to experience the same jeopardy. Some studies show that if your twin is depressed, there is a high percentage that you will experience the same illness. People of similar genetic makeup show similar vulnerabilities if especially the people are angry. They are likely to experience some mood swings and unstable emotion that lead to stress.

Another cause is drug abuse in some people. Some individuals take hard drugs that affect their mentality. Such personnel may change from a happy individual to a stressed character. Some medications have impacts like hallucinations, sedation, stimulation, and other effects that increase their anxiety and personality disorders. Hence such fellows will anticipate of an illusion and unrealistic goals if otherwise they are not attained thy quickly get depressed. Intoxication affects your rational beliefs and values and makes you moody, such that you are stressed due to less irritation.

Some medical conditions, like chronic diseases, put one under trauma. Such illness has painful ordeals and events. Moreover, they cause stigma to your beloved ones. Therefore, the victims view themselves as a deadweight to the family where the end-results being losing their self-esteem and feeling miserable. If you have a chronic disease like stroke, you will think others are doing more for you, which is unnecessary. Therefore, you will likely feel heartened and stressed. Consequently, one will be miserable and hopelessness.

The environmental conditions that surround you may lead to distress. Imagine being surrounded by assaultive parents, poverty conditions, or your family is regarded as an outcast. That atmosphere you are living makes one feel unappreciated. Some instances of early childhood trauma can cause depression. Take a situation a child being assaulted, that scar will probably remain with him or her he rest of their lives.

Signs Of Depression

Depression occurs in diverse, which means it occurs in very many ways. Being anxious or having unstable emotions are some of the renowned personality disorders. Imagine the emotional impact one gets after watching your loved one feeling depressed.it is, therefore, a hurtful situation. The consequences are destructive, which can even result in the individual committing suicide.

For a proper treatment of such victims, it is wise to know the type of depression one is experiencing. It is advisable to visit a clinic as soon as you realize you are experiencing some sorrows disorders. Visit the therapist as early as possible because depression is manageable at an early stage. When it is at its late-stage, it develops to become a chronic condition that puts one under pressure of health complication. Recognizing the type of depression, you are suffering from is essential because the psychiatrist will know the kind of therapeutically program to put you through. The following are some of the types of this illness.

The first type is major depressive disorder. It is the commonly known type of depression because it affects many people in society. It exhibits the typical symptoms that are accustomed to stressful reactions. These emotions involve the feeling of sadness, hopelessness, emptiness, low self-esteem, and loss of interest in major recreational activities. These symptoms are easily recognizable to a patient, and one should seek medical attention as early as possible. This disorder falls under two main categories, which are atypical depression and, melancholic type. The atypical ones always anxious therefore they eat and sleep a lot, and the melancholic beings tend to suffer from insomnia and guiltiness

There is this type of stress which is resistant the antidepressant drugs. This kind of condition is referred to as the treatment of resistant depression. You can administer any medications to this patient, but still, they are not working. They always have unknown causes where their most prominent suspects are the genetic, or environmental causatives. For one to treat those victims, psychotherapy is recommended for one to assess the reason for that moody feeling. You may also administer different types of antidepressants to establish the medicine that heals that person.

Other people who are not healed quickly from significant depression experience the subsyndromal condition. This menace involves one experiencing many melancholic disorders. In simple one is engrossed with different symptoms showing varying characteristics. You may experience melancholic and at the same time, atypical illness. The physician must be quick to detect this condition because if the patient is affected by many sicknesses, chances of healing are less.

The persistent depressive disorder involves a state of stubborn symptoms. What does it mean by them being stubborn? It means that the syndrome is continuous over time. The syndromes seem to restructure themselves where if one sign is treated, it changes and reforms to terminal disorder. Such complications involve sleeping problems, fatigue, loss of appetite, and many other conditions. The best thing for a psychiatrist to diagnose such a patient is by combining both psychotherapy and medicinal diagnosis.

Depression due to diseases is another type. Some of the chronic illnesses cause stigma to the victims. Think of how you would react if tested HIV positive, cancer, or any other fatal diseases. 'I will kill myself,' 'everybody will laugh at me and despise me.' These are your probable thoughts you would experience if told the bad news. Feelings of loneliness, regret, and guiltiness will eat you strike on you like a hungry lion.

Substance intake depression is a major one attributed to the intoxicants. Intoxication comes from people indulging in drugs and alcohol. The results were those people hallucinating or do unusual things. They will, therefore, find other people do not agree to those deeds, hence feel emotionally discouraged. Some end up in crimes and theft to buy those drugs. These substances change your mood, loss of concern on pleasurable practices, and feeling empty always. Specialized rehabs centers are useful in healing those patients.

It is every parent's joy to have a baby. However, did you know that for some people, child giving can be stressful? Probably this amazes you, but it is a fact. Some mothers change their attitude after giving birth because there is a change in hormones, fatigue, or fear of raising a child. Fathers, in their part, can change their mood when they feel their workload will be increased. Consequently, some folks become stressful.

What Is Anxiety?

Anxiety in and of itself is not a problematic emotion, as virtually everyone experiences some degree of anxiety in their lives. You may feel anxious about being late to work, or about having a first date with someone that you are really attracted to, and this anxiety could even lead to symptoms like worry, shakiness, or sweating. In situations like these, anxiety is fairly common and is not considered to be problematic or anything to worry about. However, not everyone experiences healthy levels of anxiety when their anxious responses are being triggered by the world around them. Instead, some people experience intense and overwhelming reactions that essentially hijack their minds and prevent them from rationally or reasonably working their way through their anxious experiences.

When you begin experiencing clinical anxiety, the natural symptoms of your anxiety begin to increase significantly. Instead of just experiencing a heightened but still manageable sense of anxiety, your symptoms begin to become unmanageable and overwhelming. People who are experiencing anxiety disorder are believed to have an overactive fight or flight response, which can trigger excessive responses to their original trigger or stressor. For example, the idea of taking a bus by themselves through the city they've lived in all their lives may trigger a full-blown panic attack if they are living with an anxiety disorder. Alternatively, the idea of going to a busy public place might trigger intense feelings of discomfort and stress such as nausea, high blood pressure, and intrusive thoughts. Anxiety disorder is not always characterized by panic attacks, but also by how intense the anxious response to a trigger is, and how easy (or not) it is for the person suffering to regain control over their symptoms.

The understanding as to why anxiety develops this way in certain people is not entirely understood, though there are many reasons as to why certain people will experience anxiety. For example, if a person experiences something that was particularly traumatic or stressful, their anxious response to triggers that stimulate the memory of those challenging experiences might cause anxiety. This type of stimuli can also trigger PTSD, so it is important that if this is what has caused anxiety, you are clear as to whether it is truly anxiety that is being dealt with or if it has progressed to PTSD.

It is also believed that consistent exposure to stress and overwhelm can cause anxiety in people, which can escalate to problematic anxiety over time if they are not able to relax their minds. This likely happens from consistent exposure to cortisol and adrenaline, which are the two hormones responsible for generating feelings of stress and anxiety in people who are experiencing them. Alternatively, being in a volatile relationship with someone can also result in someone experiencing anxiety as they may be trained by their abuser to live "on edge" all the time. This anxiety is used to the advantage of the abuser who relies on their victim to be anxious all the time so that they can easily swing them off balance and abuse them further, without having the anxious victim fight back.

There are truly many reasons as to why a person may develop anxiety, but regardless of how it has developed, problematic anxiety can be troublesome and challenging to ward off. It is believed that more than 40 million people live with anxiety worldwide. Living with anxiety can be life-changing, as it can cause negative consequences in virtually every area of your life if it becomes overwhelming or out of control. For that reason, it is important that anyone who is experiencing anxiety seeks support in dealing with their symptoms so that they can hopefully be treated and resume living a normal life.

How Anxiety Affects People Who Live with It

Anxiety impacts people in different ways, which is why it can be so challenging to deal with as not every case is the same. The symptoms of anxiety can vary depending on each individual case, so identifying anxiety in yourself and knowing when it has become problematic ultimately depends on your personal feeling towards your symptoms. If you feel like you truly cannot get them under control by yourself or like they are negatively impacting your quality of life, chances are, you are dealing with problematic anxiety that needs to be treated properly.

If you are experiencing overwhelming anxiety on an ongoing basis, you might find that you are constantly feeling restless and overwhelmed even when there are no real reasons for you to feel anxious. This feeling of restlessness may come and go randomly for no apparent reason, or it may be constant if you are dealing with a more advanced case of problematic anxiety disorder. When you feel this restlessness, it may feel like every little thing can lead to you having a full-blown panic attack or intense anxiety developing around things that are seemingly minor. For example, you may be driving in your car and have the need to pass a slow driver and the act of switching lanes and passing that slow driver may result in you experiencing intense anxiety. Or maybe you are sitting on your couch and you hear a loud bang from your family in the other room and your heart rate skyrockets and you have a momentary feeling like you need to run and save yourself. These types of restlessness and responses can be extremely overwhelming and problematic and can leave you feeling like you constantly have to be prepared to have an intense response to a minor thing because it feels uncontrollable.

In addition to intense responses, you may also feel constant feelings of worrying thoughts in your mind, even if you cannot logically back up your worry with rational or reasonable reasons as to why. You may feel like you are constantly worried about things, even if you can logically understand why these feelings of worry are invalid or unlikely to ever manifest as being true. Every time you do have a reason to worry, then you might find yourself having an intense stress-related response because you were already in a heightened state of worry in the first place. As a result, it may feel like you are never able to relax and experience rest or calm because you are constantly overwhelmed and stressed out.

Due to your constant state of anxiety and worry, you may also find yourself being highly irritable and moody. It is actually not uncommon for people with anxiety to also experience intense anger, which is essentially a natural "fight" response from the fight or flight mode. You may find that in most cases you want to run away, but in cases where you cannot or where you feel like you are caught by surprise instead, you get angry. You might find yourself yelling, arguing with others, or simply holding onto feelings of intense anger and resentment on an ongoing basis because of the anxiety disorder that you live with.

Other symptoms of anxiety include concentration difficulties and sleep difficulties. As a result of your body constantly producing so much cortisol and adrenaline, it may feel like you are having a hard time paying attention or making up your mind about things. Engaging in basic conversations may be challenging and it may feel like you cannot stay focused on one task for longer than a few minutes at a time. You may also find like your stress leaks over into your sleep and that you cannot sleep soundly each night, making it challenging for you to feel well rested. Alternatively, you may find yourself so stressed out that all you want to do is sleep because it feels as though your time spent sleeping is the only peaceful time that you have. The constant stress may make it feel like you are chronically exhausted, whether you have slept too much or too little, which can leave you feeling uncomfortable and frustrated all the time.

Recognizing Anxiety in Other People

If your loved one is experiencing anxiety, the signs of their anxiety and the symptoms they experience will be fairly simple to identify. Typically, you can tell if someone else is experiencing anxiety based on their mannerisms and the way that they approach the world around them. If someone is experiencing anxiety, typically they will show it in their body language, their verbal language, and their actions, thoughts, and decisions. If your loved one is experiencing anxiety, it is important that you take the time to understand what they are going through and have compassion for them and their experiences, as anxiety can be a challenging thing for anyone to navigate. Having your acceptance and understanding around their experiences are going to be extremely helpful not only in allowing them to manage their own emotional well-being but also in helping you both manage your relationship together.

A big sign that your friend or loved one is living with anxiety is that they seem on edge all the time. Their body may seem jittery or they may fidget a lot when they are in a situation that is making them uncomfortable and it may seem as though their jitters or fidgeting are uncontrollable. It is likely that your friend does not even know that they are doing this, but instead, they do it subconsciously as they try to deal with their growing energy inside of them that is telling them that there is something wrong. They may also seem jumpy or like they scare easy, which can make it seem like they are constantly living in a state of fear. This may or may not be obvious, depending on how high functioning they are alongside their anxiety.

Another common sign that your loved one is living with anxiety is the complaint of aches and pains, especially when it comes to complaints around chest pains. In some situations, these may be indicative of a larger problem, but in people with anxiety, chest pains are extremely common and do not typically have any medical reason behind why they are happening. If your loved one's pulse is racing and they start experiencing chest pains as a result of this, chances are, they are experiencing fairly intense anxious responses and they need to seek professional help if they have not already.

While some people with anxiety have what is known as "high functioning anxiety" and are able to hide their symptoms, others are not able to and will openly voice their fears or concerns around things in their life. Often, their fears or concerns will seem rather grandiose or misplaced, making those around them wonder why they are so afraid of something that is seemingly small. Even if they are high functioning, they will likely voice their fears or concerns except they will likely do it in a way that makes their fears seem smaller than they actually are. Often, they will voice these feelings in passing, try to minimize them with their language, or voice them as if they are a joke so that they can brush it off if anyone asks them if they are serious about how they are feeling.

Another common sign that can easily be seen by yourself or others who are observing your loved one who may be experiencing anxiety is the need to have things done in a very specific way. People who are anxious often find that they need to have some form of control over everything around them as this supports them in feeling like there will be no "surprises" or unexpected turn of events. By making sure that the actions they take and sometimes the actions of those around them are done in a very specific way, the person with anxiety feels like they are in control over their lives. Anytime something does not go according to "plan", they may seem very distraught and overwhelmed, possibly having a large emotional reaction to the experience that may even seem beyond reasonable. If this is happening, there is a very likely chance that your loved one is experiencing anxiety and is not attempting to be controlling or inconsiderate, but instead is simply trying to control themselves and their experience. In other words, this is not their way of trying to make you feel bad, but instead, it is their way of trying to make themselves feel good.

How Anxiety Was Treated in the Past

Unlike depression, the historical treatments of anxiety were much less cruel and gruesome. In the past, anxiety was believed to be a disturbance of ones' inner peace and it was believed that they required therapies like meditation and prayer to relieve themselves of these disturbances. Ancient Greek Stoics believed that anxiety was a disturbance of the emotional mind, which was believed to be in direct opposition of the development to the rational thinking mind. They believed that through stoicism and other mindfulness development practices, people could overcome their anxiety and live a mentally free and sound life. People who were unable to manage their anxiety were believed to be mentally weak and unevolved, as they were succumbing to the emotions of their emotional mind and struggling to "harness the power of their rational mind."

During Sigmund Freud's time, Freud described anxiety as having been a buildup of sexual energies which would result in people having too much energy pent up in their body. Without releasing that energy, Freud believed that people would suffer from panic attacks and anxiety, which to his understanding was how the energy was manifesting since it was not being expelled through coitus. According to Freud, people who were suffering anxiety needed to engage in more pleasurable and satisfying sexual lives in order to help them relieve their energy to avoid having further implications with their anxiety disorder.

At a later point in history, psychologists started to believe that anxiety was something that we were conditioned to experience by our ancestors based on their own need to fight for survival. Through this understanding, the earliest stages of modern behavioral therapies began to be applied to individuals suffering from anxiety to support them in treating their anxiety. The common belief was that we needed to continually implement behavioral changes in each succeeding generation to ensure that we were passing down positive changes to the following generations.

Signs Of Anxiety

There are common anxiety symptoms that individuals experience when it comes to feelings, thoughts, physical sensation, and in terms of behaviors. It is vital to remember that anxiety is a highly subjective emotion, and people experience it differently. This means that different people may not experience the same symptoms. Each individual will also experience anxiety symptoms at a different intensity. Symptoms of anxiety can be physical, behavioral, and cognitive.

Physical symptoms of anxiety

Physical symptoms of anxiety focus on how we experience anxiety in our bodies.

A racing heart

Your heart rate is controlled by the sympathetic nervous system. More cortisol and adrenaline hormones are released by the adrenal glands when you are dealing with something stressful. As a result, receptors in the heart respond by increasing the heartbeat. Increased heartbeat leads to more blood getting pumped into the muscles. This prepares you to attack or escape from the threat. In the case of anxiety, such a racing heart can put in a vicious cycle of nervousness.

Shortness of breath

Oxygen is taken around your body by the blood. When responding to a stressful situation, more oxygen is needed in your cells to be able to deal with such a situation. Your breathing, therefore, increases to provide the extra oxygen. Breathing too quickly makes your oxygen and carbon dioxide balance to get out of whack, and you begin to breathe with your belly.

Feeling exhausted

This is a situation where you feel fatigued most of the time. This happens when your body stays on high alert due to the increased level of stress hormones. Staying on an anxiety-activated mode can be very draining hence the constant fatigue.

Lack of sleep

An anxious person sometimes finds it very difficult to fall asleep. He cannot stay asleep, and he ends up having a restless sleep that is not enough. This happens due to high levels of hormones like cortisol and adrenaline, which make it difficult for someone to fall asleep at night.

These hormones put your body in a buzzing state where it can't relax a bit and rest. Anxiety is also associated with a cycle and a series of thought that cannot allow someone to sleep.

Muscle ache

As part of responding to threat, due to being in an anxiety-activated mode, your muscles say in a tense state. They stay rigidly strained for an extended period, and they begin to ache. This leads to pain in the neck, back, and shoulders. Muscles may also tense up to the head, which can lead to and headache.

Sweaty palms

Sweating profoundly is a common anxiety side effect. Sweat glands in the whole body get influenced by the sympathetic nervous system when it is in an active mode. Apocrine organs which are on the parts with a lot of hair begin to release milky fluid due to perspiration induced by anxiety, which makes your palms to smell bad.

Hard swallowing

Anxiety makes the throat tight, and one begins to feel as if there is something stuck in it. It is called Globus Sensation, and the reason as to why it happens is unknown and can worsen the anxious situation by making you feel like you are enough lacking air.

Here is a full list of all the physical symptoms of anxiety:

- A feeling of restlessness. This is when one feels keyed up or on edge
- Feeling choked or breath shortens
- Sweating on palms
- Faster heartbeats or racing heart
- Chest discomfort or chest pains
- Trembling, feeling shaky and muscle tensions
- Diarrhea and nausea
- Stomach butterflies
- Feeling faint or dizziness
- Hot flashes and chills
- Tingling sensations or numbness
- An exaggerated startle response
- Sleep disturbance and fatigue

These symptoms come due to physiological alterations that occur in the body due to fight-or-fright response.

However, our bodies do not differentiate between a real and in the surrounding, and an imagined or anticipated threat in the future. That is, our bodies do not differentiate between fear and anxiety.

For people who panic, the above symptoms are common and familiar. Remember that you do not have to develop a full-blown anxiety disorder to have any of these symptoms. For these symptoms to be taken mean that a person has a disorder unless they get to a certain level of intensity, frequency and time duration where they cause immense distress and begin to affect the wellbeing of that person and interfere with his normal functioning.

Behavioral symptoms of anxiety

These refer to what a person does or doesn't do when they are anxious. They reflect the attempts to try to cope with aspects of anxiety which feel unpleasant. Typical behavioral symptoms to anxiety may include:

• Avoidance behaviors: a person will try to avoid the situations that produce anxiety. If a person is anxious in social gatherings, he will try to refrain from going to social events where they will be required to socialize with others. If such a person is afraid of an elevator, such a person will avoid the elevator and take the staircase.

- Escaping: a person will try to escape from an anxiety-producing situation. For example, if a person is afraid of passing in a place where there are big crowds of people, that person will try to escape from such a place, like a crowded lecture hall

- Engaging in unhealthy activities: some people may get into risk and self-destructive behaviors such as drinking excess alcohol or drug abuse to try to deal with the anxiety.

- Limiting one's scope: some people will feel pressed to limit their scope of normal activities so that they can reduce the overall anxiety that they feel due to being in a certain place or situations. They may choose to remain at the comfort of their house and home area.

- Attachment to a person or object of safety: a person with anxiety may only feel safe with a particular person or about a particular object. They may refuse to go out or away from home or to other places such as school so that they stay with their person or object they feel comfortable with. They will not want to be separated from such person or object.

The problem is that these coping symptoms worsen with time and maintain an anxiety disorder.

Emotional symptoms of anxiety

Basically, anxiety is an emotion, but it produces various feelings. These feelings become emotional symptoms. They include:

•   Apprehension: a feeling that something bad or unpleasant is going to happen in the future.

•   Distress: being sorrowful and in distressing emotional pain.

•   Dread: regarding something or someone with great awe and reverence.

•   Nervousness: you get to the point where you are not mentally settled.

•   Feeling overwhelmed: one begins to feel defeated and unable to accomplish

•   Panic: Grabbed by a sensation of fear that is so dominant to prevent reason and logical thinking.

•   Uneasiness: feeling uncomfortable with someone or a situation

•   Fear this a feeling introduced by perceived danger or threat that occurs in certain circumstances.

- Worry: This is feeling troubled by actual or potential problems

- Jumpiness or edginess: this is getting a vague unpleasant emotion in anticipation of some misfortunes.

Most of the times, people are unable to describe their emotions. This includes both adults and children. It is common to hear something say that they don't know how they feel when asked to describe their experience for some assistance. To most people, the emotional aspect of anxiety brings great distress. All the same, the other aspects of anxiety, such as physical reactions cause great disturbances in terms of their normal functions and wellbeing.

Cognitive symptoms of anxiety

Quite often, when we feel anxious, we usually have thought running through our minds, whether we know it or not. Even without anxiety, thousands of thoughts still run through our minds every day. When we experience anxiety, the kind of thoughts that run through our minds is worry thoughts. These thoughts may vary depending on the situation and the individual facing that situation. The common ones include:

1.   A person with social anxiety worries that their anxiety will be obvious and that other people will notice it and judge them. Negatively. They fear being taking as unattractive, stupid, and boring.

2.   They fear incapacitation. They feel that anxiety will make them lose control of the situation. They think that they will not be able to make it due to obsessive-compulsive disorder. The person thinks that they end up being a pedophile, although there is no evidence of it.

3.   A person with a generalized anxiety disorder will worry that their periodic worrying will harm them. It is also paradoxical that they believe worry is important for preparedness and avoidance of mistakes.

4.   Overestimation. A person with anxiety tends to overestimate the possibility of negative things coming to happen, but underestimate their capability to coping with these events when they come. For example, they underestimate their ability to be able to cope when they fall out with a friend.

5.   Anxiety makes a person lose confidence in themselves and feel stupid. They become nothing of themselves, and their thoughts get rigid or stuck.

These worrisome thoughts may vary depending on the anxiety disorder at stake or the person's history of anxiety.

Psychological symptoms of anxiety

They may include:

- Concentration problems, or inability to stay on a task

- Memory difficulties

- Hopelessness, loss of appetite, lethargy, and other depression symptoms.

At the heart of abnormal anxiety is the incorrect cognitive assessment of a situation. This means that one man overestimates the quantity of threat in a given challenge, and underestimate one's potential to cope with the challenge.

The cost of anxiety

Anxiety comes at a cost. These symptoms may take their toll on someone and deny them opportunities in life. When anxiety remains unidentified and untreated, its cost on someone can be quite high.

1.   Lost opportunities: some who has anxiety in social situations will end up losing social and work-related opportunities due to shyness. Such a person cannot stand out. Hence they will stay at their social corner and watch opportunities as they slip through their hands.

2.   Failed relationships: due to the fear of asserting oneself, a person with anxiety will end up maturing dysfunctional relationships

3.   Health problems: health-related problems such as jaw disorders, grinding of teeth, headaches, and irritable bowels syndrome will take a tall on someone with anxiety.

4.   Drugs and alcohol problems: in an attempt to deal with their unpleasant feelings, some people will end up indulging in excessive drinking of alcohol and other forms of drug abuse to drown their sorrows.

5.   Absenteeism: in an attempt to avoid situations that produce anxiety, some people will end up refusing to go work, poor performance at work, poor productivity, and they may even lose their jobs.

6. Suicide: due to embarrassment and low self-esteem, which comes as a result of anxiety, some people may begin to hate themselves and commit suicide.

The Relation Between Vagus Nerve And Depression

There is developing proof that inflammation can intensify or even offer ascent to burdensome side effects. The inflammatory response is a key part of our insusceptible framework. At the point when our bodies are attacked by microscopic organisms, infections, poisons, or parasites, the insusceptible framework initiates cells, proteins, and tissues, including the cerebrum, to assault these intruders. The principle technique is to stamp the harmed body parts, so we can give more consideration to them. Nearby inflammation makes the harmed parts red, swollen, and hot. At the point when the damage isn't confined, at that point, the framework ends up aggravated. These ace inflammatory variables offer ascent to "affliction practices." These incorporate physical, psychological and social changes. Normally, they wiped out individual encounters languor, weakness, slow response time, psychological impedances, and loss of craving. This star grouping of changes that happen when we are wiped out is versatile. It constrains us to get more rest to mend and stay disconnected so as not to spread diseases.

Be that as it may, a drawn-out inflammatory response can unleash ruin in our bodies and can put us in danger of depression and different sicknesses. There is a lot of proof cementing the connection between inflammation and depression. For instance, markers of inflammation are raised in individuals who experience the ill effects of depression contrasted with non-discouraged ones. Additionally, markers of inflammation can anticipate the seriousness of burdensome manifestations. An investigation that analyzed twins who offer 100 percent of similar qualities found that the twin who had a higher CRP fixation (a proportion of inflammation) was bound to create depression five years after the fact.

Specialists saw that their malignancy and Hepatitis C patients treated with IFN-alpha therapy (increments inflammatory response) likewise experienced depression. This treatment expanded the arrival of genius inflammatory cytokines, which offered ascend to lost hunger, rest aggravation, anhedonia (loss of joy), subjective impedance, and self-destructive ideation. The pervasiveness of depression in these patients was high. These outcomes add assurance to the inflammation story of depression.

Ensuing cautious investigations demonstrated that the expansion in the commonness of depression in patients treated with IFN-alpha was not just in light of the fact that they were wiped out. Utilizing a basic technique for infusing sound subjects with invulnerable framework intruders, specialists discovered higher paces of burdensome side effects during the ones which were presented contrasted with the fake treatment gathering. The subjects who were initiated to have an inflammatory response whined of indications, for example, negative state of mind, anhedonia, rest unsettling influences, social withdrawal, and intellectual weaknesses.

The connection between inflammation and depression is much increasingly strong for patients who don't react to flow antidepressants. Studies have demonstrated that treatment-safe patients will, in general, have raised inflammatory components circling at gauge than the responsive ones. This is clinically significant; a clinician can use a measure like CRP levels, which are a piece of a routine physical, to foresee the restorative response to antidepressants. In one examination, they found that expanded degrees of an inflammation particle preceding treatment anticipated poor response to antidepressants.

There are ecological components that reason inflammation and in this way, lift hazard for depression: stress, low financial status, or an agitated youth. Additionally, a raised inflammatory response prompts expanded affectability to stretch. The impact has been accounted for in numerous investigations in mice. For instance, mice that have gone under ceaseless flighty pressure have more elevated levels of inflammation markers. Strikingly, there are singular contrasts that make a few mice progressively impervious to push, in this way starting a more quiet safe response.

Depression is a heterogeneous disorder. Every patient's battle is extraordinary given their youth, hereditary qualities, and the affectability of their resistant framework, other existing real diseases, and their flow status in the public eye. Being on the disadvantageous finish of these measurements bothers our safe framework and causes incessant inflammation. The cerebrum is extremely responsive to these flowing inflammatory markers and starts "infection conduct." When the inflammation is drawn out by stressors or different vulnerabilities, the affliction conduct moves toward becoming depression.

Reasons for anxiety

Anxiety might be brought about by a state of mind, a physical condition, the effects of medications, or a blend of these. The specialist's underlying assignment is to check whether your anxiety is a manifestation of another ailment.

Current research on Anxiety Disorder

Much research is being done into what causes anxiety disorders. Specialists trust it includes a mix of components, including qualities, diet, and stress.

Investigations of twins recommend that hereditary qualities may assume a job. For instance, an investigation announced in plos ONE Trusted Source recommends the RBFOX1 quality might be engaged with the improvement of anxiety-related conditions, for example, summed up anxiety disorder. The creators accept that both hereditary and nongenetic variables have an influence.

Certain pieces of the cerebrum, for example, the amygdala and hippocampus, are additionally being considered. Your amygdala is a little structure somewhere inside your cerebrum that procedures risk. It cautions the remainder of your mind when there are indications of risk. It can trigger a dread and anxiety response. It appears to have an influence in anxiety disorders that include dread of explicit things, for example, felines, honey bees, or suffocating.

Your hippocampus may likewise influence your danger of building up an anxiety disorder. It's a locale of your cerebrum that is associated with putting away recollections of undermining occasions. It seems, by all accounts, to be littler in individuals who've encountered kid misuse or served in battle.

What causes anxiety disorders?

Anxiety is a psychological wellness condition that can cause sentiments of stress, dread, or pressure. For certain individuals, anxiety can likewise cause fits of anxiety and extraordinary physical side effects, similar to chest torment.

The definite reasons for anxiety disorders are obscure. As indicated by the National Institute of Mental Health, specialists accept that a mix of hereditary and ecological variables may assume a job. Cerebrum science is likewise being concentrated as a conceivable reason. The zones of your mind that control your dread response might be included.

Anxiety disorders frequently happen close by other psychological wellness conditions, for example, substance misuse and depression. Numerous individuals attempt to facilitate the side effects of anxiety by utilizing liquor or different medications. The help these substances give is brief. Liquor, nicotine, caffeine, and different medications can exacerbate an anxiety disorder.

Anxiety disorders are unimaginably normal. They influence an expected 40 million individuals in the United States, as indicated by the Anxiety and Depression Association of America.

What causes anxiety and anxiety disorders can be muddled. Almost certainly, a blend of components, including hereditary qualities and ecological reasons, assume a job. In any case, plainly a few occasions, feelings, or encounters may make side effects of anxiety start or may aggravate them. These components are called triggers.

Anxiety triggers can be distinctive for every individual, except numerous triggers, are normal among individuals with these conditions. A great many people discover they have numerous triggers. Be that as it may, for certain individuals, anxiety assaults can be activated for reasons unknown by any stretch of the imagination.

Therefore, it's imperative to find any anxiety triggers that you may have. Distinguishing your triggers is a significant advance in overseeing them. Continue perusing to find out about these anxiety triggers and what you can do to deal with your anxiety.

What are the anxiety triggers

Health Issues

A wellbeing analysis that is annoying or troublesome, for example, malignancy or a constant sickness, may trigger anxiety or exacerbate it. This kind of trigger is groundbreaking on account of the prompt and individual sentiments it produces.

You can help lessen anxiety brought about by medical problems by being proactive and drawn in with your primary care physician. Conversing with a specialist may likewise be valuable, as they can enable you to figure out how to deal with your feelings around your analysis.

Medications

Certain remedy and over-the-counter (OTC) medications may trigger indications of anxiety. That is on the grounds that dynamic fixings in these medications may make you feel uneasy or unwell. Those emotions can set off a progression of occasions in your brain and body that may prompt extra side effects of anxiety.

Prescriptions that may trigger anxiety include:

- Birth control pills

- Cough and blockage medications

- Weight misfortune medications

Converse with your PCP about how these medications make you feel and search for an elective that doesn't trigger your anxiety or decline your side effects.

Caffeine

Numerous individuals depend on their morning cup of joe to wake up; however, it may really trigger or exacerbate anxiety. As per one investigation in 2010Trusted Source, individuals with frenzy disorder and social anxiety disorder are particularly touchy to the anxiety-inciting effects of caffeine.

Work to curtail your caffeine admission by substituting noncaffeinated alternatives at whatever point conceivable.

Skipping Suppers

When you don't eat, your glucose may drop. That can prompt anxious hands and a thundering stomach. It can likewise trigger anxiety.

Eating adjusted suppers is significant for some reasons. It furnishes you with vitality and significant supplements. In the event that you can't set aside a few minutes for three suppers per day, solid tidbits are an extraordinary method to anticipate low glucose, sentiments of nervousness or fomentation, and anxiety. Keep in mind, nourishment can influence your disposition.

Negative Reasoning

Your mind controls quite a bit of your body, and that is positively valid with anxiety. When you're vexed or baffled, the words you state to yourself can trigger more prominent sentiments of anxiety.

On the off chance that you will, in general, utilize a lot of negative words when considering yourself, figuring out how to refocus your language and sentiments when you start down this way is useful. Working with an advisor can be fantastically useful with this procedure.

Budgetary Concerns

Stresses over setting aside cash or having an obligation can trigger anxiety. Sudden bills or cash fears are triggers, as well.

Figuring out how to deal with these sorts of triggers may need looking for expert support, for example, from a monetary guide. Feeling you have a buddy and a guide in the process may facilitate your worry.

Gatherings Or Get-Togethers

In the event that a room brimming with outsiders doesn't seem like fun, you're not the only one. Occasions that expect you to make casual chitchat or associate with individuals you don't know can trigger sentiments of anxiety, which might be analyzed as a social anxiety disorder.

To help facilitate your stresses or unease, you can continually bring along a friend when conceivable. But at the same time, it's critical to work with an expert to discover methods for dealing with stress that make these occasions increasingly sensible in the long haul.

Struggle

Relationship issues, contentions, differences — these contentions would all be able to trigger or compound anxiety. On the off chance that contention especially triggers you, you may need to learn compromise systems. Additionally, converse with an advisor or other emotional well-being master to figure out how to deal with the sentiments these contentions cause.

Stress

Day by day stressors like congested driving conditions or missing your train can cause anybody anxiety. Yet, long haul or constant pressure can prompt long haul anxiety and compounding manifestations, just as other medical issues.

Stress can likewise prompt practices like skipping dinners, drinking liquor, or not getting enough rest. These elements can trigger or intensify anxiety, as well.

Treating and avoiding pressure regularly requires getting the hang of methods for dealing with stress. A specialist or advocate can enable you to figure out how to perceive your wellsprings of stress and handle them when they become overpowering or hazardous.

Open Occasions Or Exhibitions

Open talking, talking before your chief, performing in a challenge, or even simply perusing so anyone might hear is a typical trigger of anxiety. In the event that your activity or diversions require this, your primary care physician or advisor can work with you to learn approaches to be increasingly agreeable in these settings.

Additionally, uplifting comments from companions and associates can enable you to feel increasingly good and sure.

Individual Triggers

These triggers might be hard to distinguish, yet a psychological well-being authority is prepared to enable you to recognize them. These may start with a smell, a spot, or even a tune. Individual triggers remind you, either intentionally or unknowingly, of an awful memory or awful accident in your life. People with post-awful pressure disorder (PTSD) as often as possible experience anxiety triggers from ecological triggers.

Distinguishing individual triggers may require some serious energy, yet it's significant so you can figure out how to conquer them.

Symptoms Of Vagus Nerve Inflammation

The vagus nerve may dysfunction when it is exposed to extremely stressful conditions. Sometimes, you may not be able to tell when the nerve is dysfunctional. Normally, the symptoms associated with vagus nerve dysfunction are also associated with other conditions. You may be fooled to think that you are suffering from a different infection, yet it is due to nerve damage. We have observed that the vagus nerve supports several activities and that all the activities are vital in your daily routine. A slight dysfunction of the nerve can put most of these activities to a halt or may affect the way you function.

Vagus nerve stress can happen at any time or any day. As we delve deeper, we will be looking at environmental and social factors that can stress your vagus nerve. Knowing that the nerve can be stressed should raise the alarm on how you cater to your vagus nerve. It is necessary that you protect your nerve from any damage. All instances that may lead to the stressing of your vagus nerve must also be avoided.

Before we look at the symptoms of vagus nerve dysfunction, we should try and find out the possible ways of proving the dysfunction. As already mentioned, the symptoms for a dysfunctional vagus nerve are the same as those for a damaged nerve. The only way to be sure whether your nerve is dysfunctional or damaged is to undergo medical tests. There are several tests that can be used at a local health facility or even at home.

Doctors use the gag reflex test to determine the response of the nerve. In this test, a doctor will insert some soft tissue, maybe a cotton bud into your throat, and try to swab it on both sides. Normally, if the vagus nerve is functioning properly, the patient is supposed to feel a tickling sensation resulting in a gag. However, if the nerve has been damaged, the person may not feel anything. Other advanced tests can be used to determine the state of the vagus nerve, as we will see later on. There are different tests for diagnosing a damaged nerve, and there are individual tests that you can perform at home. However, this particular test is ideal for any individual who wishes to gain some certainty about the functioning of their vagus nerve. Before you jump into treating the nerve dysfunction, try to check the cause and make sure you have certainty that it is damaged.

Early Symptoms of Vagus Nerve Dysfunctional

There are clearly observable symptoms of vagus nerve dysfunction. However, some of these symptoms may be very diverse such that, most people never associate them with the vagus nerve. In most cases, the symptoms are associated with common conditions. If you realize that you are experiencing several of the following symptoms, it is wise to get a doctor's opinion on the health status of your vagus nerve.

• Difficulty Speaking or Loss of Voice: We have mentioned that laryngeal is the extension of the vagus nerve that extends directly to the voice box. This nerve is important in coordinating and controlling the activities of the voice box. If the nerve is damaged, muscle contraction and expansion becomes a complex duty. For this reason, any person suffering from vagus nerve damage or dysfunction is likely to suffer from voice problems.

• A Voice That Is Hoarse or Wheezy: This is still a part of the integral functions of the laryngeal. If you find out that your voice is getting horse or wheezy, the chances are that your vagus nerve has become dysfunctional. With that said, it is important to note that most people experience a wheezy voice during many instances. A simple cold could lead to a wheezy voice. This is the reason why it is important to get an opinion from the doctor before jumping into a conclusion about any symptom.

•   Trouble Drinking Liquids: We have observed that the vagus nerve plays an important role by providing motor action to some parts of the body. The most integral parts of the body where the nerve plays such a role include the pharynx. The laryngeal extension of the vagus takes action on the pharynx and stylopharyngeus muscles that affect the swallowing of food. We have determined that the vagus nerve has an effect on the muscles that determine taste and also affects the production of certain enzymes. If you start realizing that you cannot swallow drinks, the chances are that your nerve is dysfunctional.

•   Loss of the Gag Reflex: When you touch an object at the back roof of your mouth, the back muscles of the throat close automatically. This is what we refer to as the gag reflex. The gag reflex is very important since it helps a person swallow food and drinks. The reflex also plays an important role in separating the food pipe and the air pipe. In other words, if you did not have a gag reflex, the chances are that foods might find their way into the lungs. The fact that the vagus nerve controls your gag reflex means that any dysfunction of the nerve may lead to a lack of gag reflex. This option also provides one of the most reliable ways of testing your vagus nerve health. If you try touching the roof of your mouth close to the throat, you must experience an automatic closure of the throat muscles. This will give you a guarantee that your vagus nerve is still functional.

- Pain in the Ear: A branch of the vagus nerve known as auricular nerve extends to the ears. This nerve plays an important role in controlling the hearing of an individual. As a matter of fact, the auricular directly influences your sound senses. You may never be able to perceive sound well if the nerve is damaged. Pain in the ear is one of the obvious signs that the vagus nerve has been damaged. This is because the pain can only be caused by a fracture on the nerve.

- Unusual Heart Rate: The fact that the vagus nerve is linked to the heart means that any damage to the nerve may directly affect the heart rate. The cardiac extension of the vagus nerve determines the contraction of the heart muscles. This extension also helps in maintaining a steady flow of information between the heart and the brain. If the sensory nerves of the heart fail to function, the chances are that the heart may fail or may show abnormal rates. The normal heart rate is around 72 bits per second. In the case where the rate goes beyond 72, the patient should either be involved in cardiovascular exercises or the vagus nerve may be exposed to stress leading to the increased production of adrenalin.

- Abnormal Blood Pressure: We have established that the vagus nerve also affects the constriction of blood vessels. If the nerve is stimulated or under stress, it may lead to the constriction of blood vessels. Given that pressure may also lead to an increased heart rate, this simply means that over-stimulation of the nerve may cause increased blood pressure. When the heart is pumping at fast rates, yet the blood vessels have been constricted, the blood pressure is bound to increase. Such occurrences may lead to heart attacks or loss of consciousness. If you experience increased blood pressure constantly, you need to try and figure out the triggers. If your pressure is caused by vagus nerve stimulation or failure, the chances are that your nerve is malfunctioning. However, you should also remember that no all blood pressure issues are associated with the vagus nerve. Some of the blood pressure issues are associated with other lifestyle diseases.

•	Decreased Production of Stomach Acid: We have also established that the vagus nerve works in conjunction with endocrine glands to ensure that food is digested. Before endocrine glands can produce the necessary enzymes that are needed in food digestion, they must receive signals from the autonomic nervous system. The most central part of the anatomic nervous system is the vagus nerve. If you realize that you are experiencing some of the symptoms of low stomach acids such as bloating, belching, heartburns, among others, you should start observing for other signs of vagus dysfunction. These symptoms may appear in short intervals if your vagus nerve is ailing. If the nerve is completely damaged, you may experience such conditions continuously.

•	Nausea or Vomiting: Nausea and vomiting are also some of the symptoms that indicate high levels of stomach acid. If the vagus nerve is affected, it is possible to suffer from nausea and such symptoms. This is because the regulatory tissues that control the production of stomach acid are not functioning properly.

•	Abdominal Bloating or Pain: The abdomen is the final destination of the vagus nerve, with the final ending touching the spinal cord. The fact that the nerve is extended to the lower abdomen means that if it is affected, you may experience some defects in your body. Given that the nerve plays an important role in controlling stomach muscles, it can be painful, leading to abdominal pain in some people.

Advanced Symptoms of Dysfunctional

The above symptoms are general and can apply to any person who has a dysfunctional vagus nerve. However, there are cases where the nerve is severely wounded or is completely damaged. In such cases, the symptoms tend to advance. In most cases., when the damage is, to a large extent, the focus is on diseases that may result from the vagus nerve damage.

In the section above, we only focused on general symptoms that may relate to any problem to the nerve. However, as you advance to the next stages, you realize that the extent of damage to the nerve may cause some serious illnesses. There are two main diseases that doctors have linked to vagus nerve damage. We will look at these diseases in detail as we advance. In this section, we only want to look at the symptoms and how they may be a way of showing that you have a dysfunctional vagus nerve. If you cannot detect or diagnose a defective vagus nerve, you may end up living in pain for a long time without being able to tell the cause. You may even be misdiagnosed by doctors if you do not know the right information about that condition. The two main conditions that may affect a person due to a damaged vagus nerve include gastroparesis and vasovagal syncope.

Gastroparesis

Several research findings have shown that there is a direct link between gastroparesis and vagus nerve damage. This is a condition that severely affects the involuntary contraction of the digestive system. As we had mentioned, the vagus nerve, in conjunction with ANS facilitates the parasympathetic functions of the body. Some of the parasympathetic functions include involuntary contraction of the digestive system. In simple terms, when you suffer from a damaged vagus nerve, you may never enjoy parasympathetic actions of defecation. The stomach does not empty properly, and this leads to a continuous pile up of previous dirt. Some of the common symptoms of this condition include

•   Nausea or Vomiting: In the symptoms above, we mentioned nausea and vomiting. However, this case is much worse and severe. In the case of gastroparesis, the patient is unable to let out most of the food eaten. This leads to nausea and vomiting of foods long hours after eating. In normal vomiting situations, a person just vomits a few minutes after eating. However, in these advanced cases of gastroparesis, the victim is likely to vomit after very many hours of waiting.

- Loss of Appetite: Most people who suffer from gastroparesis, often eat a little food and constantly lack appetite. This condition makes a person feel full even when they are hungry. Patients suffering from this condition may either completely lack appetite or feel full after eating just a little amount. However, there are many other conditions that may still lead to a lack of appetite. Do not be quick to jump to conclusions just because a person lacks appetite. If you feel that you are suffering from a lack of appetite, investigate all the possible causes. You may also have a doctor test you for vagus nerve dysfunction.

- Acid Reflux: Acid refluxes will just occur as it is the case above. However, in this case, they will be much more severe and may be recurrent.

• Abdominal Pain or Bloating: The other direct symptom of gastroparesis is bloating and abdominal pain. The vagus nerve spreads to the lower abdomen, having an influence on your excretory and sexual organs. This means that any damage to the nerve may directly affect your sexual health or your digestive health. Such conditions will often lead to abdominal pain.

• Unexplained Weight Loss: There are several reasons why a person suffering from gastroparesis may lose weight. First, such individuals do not eat as much as they should eat. This means that the body is denied some of the essential vitamins. Further, the body does not fully digest the food consumed. In most cases, the food has to come out through vomit. Such issues often lead to a loss of weight in most patients — this a distinctive observation for the severe stage of vagus nerve damage. In the early symptoms, the patient may experience digestive complications, but they are not to the extent of affecting personal weight. In essence, those who suffer from the early stages of vagus nerve damage still have a choice to make on the types of foods they want to eat. They may still eat without vomiting. However, the stage where gastroparesis develops, it is almost impossible to manage the effects associated with eating.

- Fluctuations in Blood Sugar: If you do not eat properly, you will end up affecting your blood sugar. The human body's blood sugar is balanced by the food being processed into glucose and absorbed into the system. However, if the stomach is not in a position to digest all the food that you eat, you are likely to encounter severe shortages in energy and blood sugar.

We have mentioned that some traditional treatment methods advocate for the removal of the vagus nerve through a process known as vagotomy. In this process, part of the nerve was cut off to help patients who suffer from increased stomach ulcers. However, it was realized that this process had several side effects. One of the most severe side effects associated with the vagotomy was the development of gastroparesis. It was realized that patients who underwent the process suffered advanced symptoms only associated with this condition.

Vasovagal Syncope

It is common for the vagus nerve to overreact to stress or stimulation. In the case of an overreaction, the vagus nerve may develop a condition known as vasovagal syncope. This condition can lead to a sudden drop in heart rate and blood pressure. If a person undergoes an extreme stressing situation that directly affects the vagus nerve, the drop in pressure may result in loss of consciousness (fainting). This is the condition that is known as vasovagal syncope. It is important to remember that the vagus nerve plays a central role in stimulating several muscles in the heart that directly affect your heart rate. If the nerve is overstressed, it may lead to a slowdown in the body processes leading to this condition.

Some of the extreme pressure events that can lead to vasovagal include:

•   Exposure to Extreme Heat: Exposure to extreme heat all over sudden or for long hours may lead to excessive dilation of blood vessels. The dilation, in conjunction with the reduced pressure due to stress, may result in low blood pressure and a slow heart rate. This scenario is likely to lead to a loss of consciousness.

•   Fear of Bodily Harm: Most people react differently to emotional situations. The emotion of fear has the strongest effect on the vagus nerve. When a person is afraid, excessive levels of adrenaline are produced to start the fight or flight state of the body. In this state, the vagus nerve is under extreme pressure. If someone was to startle you in the dark, you might undergo this type of excessive pressure. This may lead to a sudden drop in blood pressure and lead to a sudden loss of consciousness. In some people, the same action may lead to increased heart rate, increased blood pressure, and body heat. It is common to see people sweating under intense fear.

•	The Sight of Blood or Having Blood Drawn: If you have fear for blood or if you fear needles, you may also undergo vasovagal syncope. This is common when a person sees blood for the first time. Since the picture blood creates a situation of intense fear, you are likely to stress the vagus nerve. This may lead to a sudden drop in blood pressure and heart rate, and as a result, lead to fainting.

•	Straining: One of the ways to detect that a person is suffering from vasovagal is by observing the strain they go through. If you find yourself straining to have bowel movements, the chances are that you are suffering from vasovagal syncope. The pressure on the vagus nerve usually affects the digestive system and may lead to reduced intestinal action.

•	Standing for a Long Time: Standing for a long time may create pressure on the vagus nerve. One of the reasons being that the upper body needs support to hold the nerve. When the neck and thorax muscles have to support themselves on the nerves for long hours, a person may experience problems in the natural flow of blood. This explains why it is common for people to faint after standing for long hours. The long hours may lead to a drop in heart rate and blood pressure and eventually lead to fainting.

What Happens If The Vagus Nerve Is Damaged?

As we have observed, it is possible that the vagus nerve can be damaged. The nerve can be damaged due to excessive pressure on the nerve or due to stress. Continuous stimulation of the nerve can lead to damage if it is not done in the right way. There are also surgical medical procedures that can lead to the nerve being cut or damaged by surgical instruments. In either case, nerve damage can cause serious problems for the patient.

If your nerve is completely damaged, you may experience some of the following problems.

• Speaking or Voice Problems: Damaged nerves can affect the voice box, which may lead to a wheezy voice or difficulty in speaking.

• Trouble Eating and Drinking: Any damage to the vagus nerve may affect how your throat muscles operate. Given that they are responsible for swallowing food, you will eventually experience problems when taking food or swallowing water. In essence, vagus nerve damage mainly affects the gag reflex. As we have already observed, the gag reflex is responsible for ensuring that the food pipe is opened up to allow the swallowing of foods as you eat.

• Loss of Hearing or Pain in the Ear: There are high chances that your hearing will be affected in case your vagus nerve gets damaged. Any damage to the vagus nerve may lead to pain in the ear, given that the nerve extends to the outermost part of the ear. The nerve is also linked directly to your eardrums. This shows that any damage to the nerve may affect your hearing ability and may lead to loss of hearing or may cause pain in the ears.

• Affected Heart Rate and Blood Pressure: When your vagus nerve is affected, you must expect significant changes in your heart rate and blood pressure. The vagus nerve is the extension of the autonomic nervous system that directly links the heart to the brain. This means that any action that may affect the vagus can directly impact on the coordination between the heart and the brain. This may cause major damage to your heart and definitely affect the heart rate. When the heart rate is affected, then the blood pressure is also affected. The blood pressure is maintained by a steady heartbeat. If the heartbeat jumps up a bit, the blood pressure also fluctuates.

- Abdominal Pains and Stomach Pains: Damage to the vagus nerve often leads to decreased stomach acids. This means that you may experience some problems with food digestion. There is a level of stomach acids that should be maintained at all times. Any damage to the vagus nerve means that the glands responsible for the production of stomach acids do not get signals that start the process of acid production. Further, any damage to the vagus nerve may also affect abdominal muscles. It is the vagus nerve in conjunction with the nervous system that stimulates the abdominal areas. The nerve is responsible for sexual arousal because it extends to all the sexual parts. The nerve sends signals that start ovulation and other sexual activities. If the nerve is damaged, the chances are that a person may experience some abdominal pains. This is particularly true in ladies.

Communication Effects of Vagus Nerve Damage

The vagus nerve affects all the sensory aspects of your body. In other words, your six senses are related to the nerve in some way. One of the senses that directly relies on the vagus nerve is your hearing. Unlike smell and taste that partially rely on the vagus nerve, the hearing sense is entirely linked to the well-being of the vagus nerve. Any damage to the nerve may lead to a variety of problems.

The auricular vagus nerve is the nerve that links the central vagus nerve from the brain with the ear. The auricular vagus never ends on the back skin of the wear, extending a variety of smaller nerves on the ear. One of the important roles played by this nerve is sensory action. In simple terms, the nerve is responsible for collecting communication senses and sending signals to the brain for interpretation. If the nerve was not in place, it would be a big problem for most people to perceive communication. Some of the problems that would occur in your communication if the vagus nerve was damaged include:

Inability to Perceive Words: We perceive words during communication, not only from our hearing but also from observation. When you look at a person, you can tell what they are saying by looking at their lips. In many ways, these observations help us link what a person is saying to their voice, making communication easy and flawless. However, in a case where the vagus nerve is completely damaged, the sensory aspect of our hearing is lost. We are unable to place a direct relationship to the voice and movements of the mouth from the other person. This brings a lot of complications in the communication process. It is important to have a clear sense when speaking to a person so that you can perceive what they are saying even when you cannot hear the words directly.

Inability to Perceive the Direction of Voices: One way that human beings maintain a clear focus in life is through the ability to sense the direction of the voice. While you may hear voices, without knowing the direction and distinctly separating one sound from another, you may be in huge trouble. The balanced sense of voices helps a person maintain stability while standing or walking. Any imbalances in the hearing aspects may cause a person to lean towards one side. If the vagus nerves in one year are damaged, this may force a person to tilt to one side, where the vagus sense is active.

Being in a position to sense the direction of a voice contributes to a large extent in the communication process. For instance, in a room where you have to communicate with several people at a go, you may not be able to function appropriately if your ears fail to sense the direction from which the sound is coming. If you work at a pace where communication flows through a chain, you may have problems when trying to link up the chain.

The most dangerous scenario in vagus nerve failure would come when you are crossing streets. Knowing the direction of sound is important in helping a person perceive warnings from cars while walking on the streets. If you do not know where a sound is coming from, you may easily be involved in road accidents. You may take longer to recognize cars coming your way, or you may easily confuse the direction of a warning sound and run directly into the same danger.

All these factors show the importance of the vagus nerve in facilitating communication. It is important to ensure that the nerve remains healthy so that it does not affect communication in any way. Failure of the nerve may lead to many problems at a personal level.

Inability to Perceive High Volumes: Another danger that a person suffering from a damaged vagus nerve faces is the inability to perceive volumes. Although the person might be able to hear, they lose the sense of detecting the volume range. This means that the patient may be exposed to very high volumes without noticing. This is a big danger given that the high volumes may lead to eardrum damage. The sensory aspect of the vagus nerve is very vital in protecting the ear from noise and high volumes. If your sensory nerves are completely damaged, you fail to differentiate sounds and volumes. The ear does not send the necessary signals to the brain. This leaves the patient exposed to dangerous situations that may lead to the damage of the eardrums and eventually cause a total loss of hearing.

If you are unable to perceive volumes, you also miss a lot in communication. When communicating with a person, you need to perceive their actions and pay attention to tonation. If a person raises their voice during an argument or a debate, you can perceive from the raised tone that the person is getting emotional. Such clues can only be detected if your nerves play the role of detecting communication flaws. If your vagus nerve is entirely damaged, you are not in a position to understand communications that result from voice variations. This is another reason why you must protect your vagus nerve from any damage.

Pain in the Ear: Another effect of the damaged vagus nerve in communication is constant pain in the ear. This does not affect your hearing as much, but continuous pain may lead to further complications. If you constantly feel pain in the ear or in the veins that extend to the ear, the chances are that your vagus nerve has been damaged. People who suffer from damaged auricular nerve usually feel pain from the ear, extending all the way to the neck. The auricular nerve links up from the lower part of your neck, this means that any damage to your ear nerves may affect your neck and your head. Damages to the vagus nerve in the ear section may lead to pain in the neck and headaches constantly. These factors affect your concentration. This type of pain may lead to hearing problems in the long run too. The patient is likely to feel as if the ears are clouded with dust. It is often difficult for the patient to perceive communications due to the pain and discomfort. Most people who suffer from damaged nerves stay in a state of discomfort and unease for a long time. When they speak, they have to strain thinking that other people may also not perceive the communication effectively.

The Response of the Body When the Nerve Damage

The vagus nerve serves a large part of our internal and external bodies. There are key body parts that will lose their sense if the vagus nerve is damaged. We have already established that the vagus nerve provides two components of sensory response. The somatic component mainly refers to the external sensory sensation provided by the nerve. The external senses of the vagus nerve are mainly felt on the skin or in the muscles. In areas of the body where the vagus nerve extends to the skin, you are able to feel a sensation associated with the nerve. A good example is an ear, where the auricular nerves extend to the surface of the ears.

The other component of sensory provided by the vagus nerve is known as the visceral sense. This mainly refers to sensations felt in the internal body organs. In essence, the vagus nerve has control over very key internal body organs and is responsible for the response of such organs during moments when the body is required to take action.

A damaged vagus nerve may affect both somatic and visceral components of the body. The sensory components provide by this nerve are not only important in keeping a person alert, but they also facilitate internal body processes. This means that the nerve plays a central role in detecting changes in the body and also enhances the production of necessary hormones. If these sensory properties of the nerve are cut off due to vagus nerve damage, it would be impossible for any person to lead a normal life. As we have observed, some of the problems associated with vagus nerve damage are due to sensory failure. For instance, in a case where a person has undergone vagotomy, the chances are that the vagus nerve may fail to stimulate intestinal glands to secret stomach acids when they are needed. As a result, a person may suffer acid reflux, vomiting, nausea, among other conditions. We have also seen that individuals who suffer from damaged vagus nerve may constantly lack appetite or vomit all the food soon after eating. All these factors are related to the fact that the glands required to secrete enzymes and acids do not get the right signal from the nervous system. Any damage to the vagus nerve may affect the following body parts and organs.

The Ear: The sense of hearing may largely be damage. This is because the auricular vagus nerve extends to the outer skin of the ear. This means that, if a person has a damaged neve, the ears may not be able to feel any sense of touch or sometimes perceive sounds. The vagus nerve to the ear extends to the ear canal. This means that the ear canal may be damaged even without a person sensing the pain. All these factors affect a person's communication, as we have seen above. If you want to maintain your hearing, you must protect your vagus nerve from damage. We have already looked at some of the causes of ear canal damage. In your efforts to try and protect your ear from getting damaged, you can use the points mentioned. We will also look at some natural ways of protecting your vagus nerve as we proceed.

Throat: The other body part that may be affected by vagus nerve damage is the throat. The vagus nerve to the ear extends to the throat. It is the vagus nerve that supports gag flex, which is an important physiological process in the body. Without gag flex, it is impossible for any person to eat and swallow food. The damage to your vagus nerve my affect throat muscles leading to failure in the mouth and actions in the mouth.

Visceral Sensation for the Larynx: The larynx (voice box) is an important organ that plays a central role in your communication. The response of this body part primarily depends on the well-being of the vagus nerve. Even if you try speaking, you may not succeed as long as your vagus nerve is completely damaged. In other words, a damaged vagus nerve may directly affect your speech. Some people who have damaged vagus nerves produce wheezy voices while others completely fail to speak. The extent to which the nerve is damaged determines the level of communication. If the damage is severe, a person may be completely inaudible when they speak.

Sensory Effect for the Esophagus: The esophageal is the extension of the vagus nerve to the esophagus. This nerve is very important in sending communications to the brain and back to the esophagus. The vagus nerve plays an important role in directing food down to the stomach. If the esophagus does not have a sensory effect, then the food swallowed may not move down to the stomach. The esophagus is always in constant constriction to help the movement of food as it is lowered into the stomach. All these movements are directly supported by the subconscious actions of the vagus nerve. If the vagus nerve is damaged, there would be a problem since a person would have to consciously strain to push the food into the stomach.

Sensory Action in the Lungs: The lungs are an integral part of your being and are part of the body that are affected by any damage to the vagus nerve. Lungs do not only help you breathe, but they also affect the flow of fresh air into the brain. The movement of fresh air into the lungs, to the brain and back out is influenced by the vagus nerve. It is the nerve that determines the rate of contraction and expansion of the blood vessels. Although such actions happen subconsciously, any damage to the vagus nerve may directly affect your breathing, leading to far-reaching effects in your normal life.

Sensory Action in the Trachea: Also known as the windpipe, the trachea is an important body organ that connects your throat to your lungs. We have mentioned that the gag reflex in your throat is responsible for the separation of food and air at the throat. You have probably have been in a position where tiny pieces of food found their way into the trachea. Even if it is a very tiny piece of food, it leads to extensive coughing and suffocation. If action is not taken in a few minutes, a person may be chocked to death. This explains how delicate the trachea can be. The vagus nerve sensory action helps to distinguish the esophagus from the trachea. Through the sensory action of the vagus nerve, foods are directly moved to the esophagus while air is directed to the trachea. The sensory action of the vagus nerve helps manipulate the trachea to help control to counter movement of fresh air in and used air out. All these aspects would be affected in case the vagus nerve is damaged. The trachea would fail to coordinated the activities that lead to easy breathing, hence creating complications.

Sensory Action to the Heart: The heart is probably the most important organ of the human body. The fact that its actions are directly coordinated by the vagus nerve sends chills on the thought of a damaged vagus nerve. The pulmonary and cardiac extensions of the vagus nerve directly coordinate the activities of the heart. Like all the other parasympathetic actions of the vagus nerve, the activities of the heart are controlled subconsciously. In other words, the vagus nerve is able to coordinate the actions of the heart without your perceptions. The key sensory activities of the vagus nerve include the contraction of heart muscles, constriction of blood veins, and the communication between the heart and the brain. All these actions can directly impact the heart rate and blood pressure, as we have already observed. Any damage to the vagus nerve may mean disruption to the regular activities carried out by the heart. Some of the regular activities carried out may stop or may adopt an irregular pattern. We have seen that overstimulation of the vagus nerve may lead to a drop in blood pressure or an increase in heart rate. If this is the case, a damaged nerve may also lead to a serious drop in heart pressure. These actions are likely to cause fainting. The case gets worse if the vagus nerve is completely damaged. In this case, a person may get into a permanent state of unconsciousness.

Sensory Action of the Digestive System: The other important body organ that can be affected by the vagus nerve is the digestive system. Although the sensory effect of the vagus nerve on the system is subconscious, it is very vital. The vagus nerve coordinates with endocrine glands to facilitate the excretion of hormones and enzymes. When a person eats, the signal from the vagus nerve in the stomach allows the excretion of necessary hormones to help in the digestion of the food. Further, the sensory activities of the vagus nerve allow movement in the small intestines. This means that, when the food gets into the intestines, the vagus nerve senses the action and prompts the movement. This movement of intestinal muscles is important in facilitating digestion and absorption of food and nutrients.

In a case where the vagus nerve has been damaged, the entire digestive system would be affected in three ways. First, the endocrine glands will not receive signals prompting the secretion of enzymes that are necessary for the digestive process. Secondly, the stomach acid levels will drop significantly, affecting the overall digestion of foods. Lastly, any damage to the vagus nerve may also affect the movements in the stomach and intestines. Any effect on the intestinal movements may affect the flow and absorption of foods. We have observed that when the vagus nerve is damaged, the walls of the intestines may not provide the necessary action. This may lead to slow absorption of foods and nutrients. In most cases, individuals who suffer from this condition may end up vomiting all the food they take. It is common for patients to lack appetite and to spend many days without visiting the washroom. It often leads to loss of weight, lack of energy, and constant fatigue. This gives us a reason to protect our vagus nerves no matter what.

Taste Sensory Glands: The vagus nerve also plays a small role in sensory glands. Although the nerve does extend to the tongue, it does take a role in the taste senses. It accounts for less than 1/3 of the taste senses. However, it does play a role in tasting and smelling foods. Smaller nerves are entrenched on the root of the tongue that facilitates tasting the foods. It is believed that these nerves also play a minor role in facilitating the production of enzymes in the mouth for food digestions.

Blood Pressure Effects Due to Nerve Damage

The blood pressure of a person is directly dependent on the heart rate and blood vessel constriction. Both of these factors are directly affected by the vagus nerve. Vagus nerve stimulation is one of the techniques that are used in treating high blood pressure and epilepsy. The reason why this approach is used is that high blood pressure can be controlled by stimulating the vagus nerve. When the nerve is damaged, it is impossible to help or control the heart rate or the constriction of blood vessels. This means that, in case of high blood pressure, there is no way of controlling it.

Protecting your vagus nerve from damage means that you protect your heart and your entire health. One of the most dangerous diseases is heart attacks. All heart-related conditions can lead to instant death if they are not well managed. For many years, medical practitioners have relied on the power of the vagus nerve to treat heart conditions such as high blood pressure. It is common for people to pass out when the blood pressure drops considerably or raises above the normal. It is, therefore, important to ensure that the vagus nerve is healthy at all times to help in controlling unfortunate instances of heart conditions.

Some of the moments when the heart rate may rise considerably include when a person is stressed or afraid of physical harm. Any mater that may threaten the life of a person may lead to an increased heart rate. Even a simple scary scene from a horror movie may drastically shift the heart rate of a person. While there are some scary factors or threats that we can avoid, it is not possible to always avoid such factors. From time to time, people are faced with threats that lead to dangerous heart conditions. People who suffer from anxiety are more likely to experience heart-racing events. If a person suffers from anxiety, they are easily scared or emotionally triggered by something that may be considered a non-issue by another person. For this reason, we must also ensure that we protect those who suffer from anxiety and depression from severe heart conditions. The only possible and safe way of offering such protection is ensuring that the vagus nerve remains healthy and functional.

We have established that overstimulation of the vagus nerve may have some severe effects on a person. It is important to ensure that even if you stimulate your vagus nerve, you use appropriate techniques. We looked at some of the artificial methods of vagus nerve stimulation that may directly impact a person. Do not use any methods of stimulation that may lead to damage or inflammation of the vagus nerve. If you desire to protect your nerve and your life as a whole, you must pay attention to less harmful techniques. There are many vagus nerve stimulation techniques that can help you protect the health of the nerve and prevent any damages that may be costly in the long run. A damaged vagus nerve can be very dangerous and may vastly affect your heart rate and blood pressure.

How To Stimulate Vagus Nerve

Natural Ways of Vagus Nerve Stimulation

Besides meditation, slow breathing, and yoga, there are other techniques of vagus nerve stimulation that are less harmful. Look at these techniques and use them to stimulate your vagus nerve when you are anxious or nervous.

Chewing Gum: Chewing gum leads to the secretion of CCK, a gut hormone that directly activates vagal impulses. This explains why people are likely to remain active for long hours while chewing gum. When a person chews gum, he/she can go for hours without taking food. This is due to the vagal impulses that CCK sends to the brain. The brain is tricked into thinking that the person is eating food. This trick can be used to reduce the sensory actions that lead to feelings of hunger in a person.

Eat High Fiber Foods: High fiber foods have also been found to be helpful in stimulating the action of the vagus nerve. Fiber foods are a good source of GLP-1, a satiating hormone that is responsible for the stimulating vagus impulses in the brain. This hormone helps slow down gut action and as a result, makes a person feel fuller for a long time. Some of the important high fiber foods include grains such as barley and peas. You can also rely on carrots, nuts, and potatoes, among others.

Tai Chi: We have already looked at tai-chi as one of the most effective ways of stimulating the vagus nerve. This is a 100% natural process since it does not involve the use of electronic gadgets. Tai-chi is known for its ability to increase heart rate variability; as a result, directly influencing the actions of the vagus nerve.

Gargling: Gargling may seem like child's play to many, but it is an important exercise that may influence your vagus nerve health. Gargling activates the vagus nerve and stimulates the gastrointestinal tract. Naturally, it is the vagus nerve that is supposed to activate the muscles behind the throat, allowing you to gargle. However, in a case where the action of the vagus nerve is slow, and the body needs some stimulation, self-induced gargling leads to the contraction of the muscles in the back of your throat, hence stimulating the vagus nerve. You can naturally stimulate your vagus nerve by gargling water before you swallow it.

Singing or Chanting: Another way of influencing the activity of your vagus nerve us through singing and chanting. Singing increases heart variability, just like it is the case with tai chi. Some of the best chants and songs include humming, mantra recitation, hymn singing, etc. These types of songs or any hyperactivity dance and song performance can influence your vagus nerve to a large extent. When you sing, you stimulate the vagus pump, which sends relaxing waves to the brain through the choir. If you chant or sing at the top of your voice, you activate the muscles behind the throat, which stimulate the vagus nerve for action.

Positive Socialization: Social relationships can make a person overcome some of the negative emotions that lead to anxiety. If you relate well with people, you are more likely to feel calm and relaxed even when the situations are tough. In one study conducted by the Michigan University Psychology Department, participants were asked to sit separately and think compassionately about their family and friends. The participants were also required to silently repeat passionate phrases such as ……..may you feel happy, may you feel safe, may you live well, etc.

Compared to those controlling the research, the participants of the exercise showed an overall increase in positive emotions such as joy, amusement, serenity, interest, among others. These changes were associated with a sense of being connected. As a result, the participants experienced improved vagal activity as observed through their heart rate variability. If you want to be genuinely happy and live well in all situations, you must learn to embrace people. Bring people together and love your life with joy.

Laughter: They say laughter is the best medicine. When it comes to taking care of your mental and social health, there is no better option than laughter. Several studies indicate that laughter is the best medicine since it stimulates the vagus nerve. One research showed that yoga laughter led to increased heart rate variability among the participants. This goes to show that the heart can be affected by your laughter. When a person laughs, the back muscles of the thought are stimulated in the same way as gargling. This stimulation leads to the activation of the vagus nerve, bringing in a feel-good sense. You can improve your vagus nerve health by getting involved in activities that promote laughter.

Vagus nerve can also be inflamed due to increased stimulation. While stimulation of the vagus nerve is something good that can help you stimulate the parasympathetic action, it can also be dangerous. If the nerve is overstimulated, the chances are that the pressure on the nerve may get excessive and lead to injuries. You must especially avoid means of vagus nerve stimulation that are not natural. Some of the artificial ways of vagus nerve stimulation that can lead to inflammation include:

PEMF

Pulsed Electromagnetic Field (PEMF) is a therapy that is often used to increase the heart rate and variability. This therapy is often used to stimulate the vagus nerve, prompting parasympathetic actions. While the use of PEMF is not harmful, continuous stimulation of the vagus nerve using this approach may lead to injuries, damage, or inflammation.

Most people use electromagnetic stimulators over the throat to naturally increase appetite. The same approach can also be used for self-stimulation and boosting bad moods. The fact that the pulsed gadget is applied directly to the brain, neck, or gut, makes it even more dangerous.

This means that the devices used in the stimulation process have to come in direct contact with a person.

At times, you may be exposed to vagus nerve stimulating machines without knowing. Before you start using any electronic stimulation devices, try to understand the principles under which it operates. While a gadget may help you by stimulation your vagus nerve during the first few days, continued stimulation may be dangerous. Continued stimulation may lead to the inflammation of the vagus nerve, which may, in turn, be costly to treat.

Probiotics

We are living in an age where people are obsessed with living their lives according to the trends. In recent years, many people have shifted to the lifestyle of taking supplements and probiotics. As to whether probiotics are good for your health or not is a subject for another day. In this section, we only look at the effects of consuming probiotics on your vagus nerve. As it turns out, consuming probiotics for long may actually affect the vagus nerve negatively.

We have already established that the nervous system is connected to the brain through the vagus nerve. This means that messing with the vagus nerve messes up with the entire system. Recent studies show that there is an effect of the gut microbiota on the brain. In other words, the probiotics you consume may find their way to the brain and affect the nervous system in its entirety.

In one animal study on mice carried out by MIT, mice supplements were enriched with probiotics. The mice that consumed the supplements experienced a positive change in GABA receptors, which were mediated by the vagus nerve. GABA receptors are vital in the brain since they help regulate mood and provide a clear connection between the brain and vagus nerve stimulation. Continuous consumption of probiotics foods means that you may be stimulating your vagus nerve even without knowing. Continuous stimulation of your nerve through such artificial methods may have an effect on your vagus nerve, leading to damage or inflammation in the long run. As much as probiotics have shown positive health benefits, they are also very effective in stimulating the vagus nerve. There is time to stimulate the nerve. Do not get used to eating probiotics daily since it may only lead to overstimulation of the nerve.

Serotonin

Serotonin is a monoamine neurotransmitter that can be consumed artificially. Although the body is fully capable of producing its natural neurotransmitters, most people prefer boosting their mental clarity by consuming artificial serotonin. Research shows that consumption of serotonin may lead to the activation of the vagus nerve through various receptors, including 5HT1A, 5-HT3, 5-HT6, among others. However, there are some receptors that may lower the activity of the vagus nerve. For instance, serotonin through the 5-HT7 receptors does reduce the activation of the vagus nerve. In simple terms, serotonin offers a mixed bag of reactions for any individual who wishes to activate their vagus nerve. This mixed outcome poses a big danger to the vagus nerve. When taking serotonin, you must be sure of the type of receptors you are targeting. The serotonin that activates the vagus nerve may still lead to inflammation. Continuous activation of the vagus nerve through artificial means only builds pressure on the nerve. When your vagus nerve is under pressure, it is likely to suffer injuries or get damaged. The final outcome of the injuries or damage includes inflammation. In case the vagus nerve is damaged, you have to use counteraction to reduce the inflammation caused by the natural healing mechanisms. It is recommended for those who take serotonin to use the 5-HTP for the purpose of increasing serotonin. However, you should take your supplements over a long period with a clear distribution of the injection sessions.

Activating Your Vagus Nerve Effortlessly

While everyone is born with different levels of vagal tone, you can have an effect on it. If your vagal tone is low, there are steps you can take to activate your vagus nerve and improve its tone. I have personally tried a large number of the activities and techniques mentioned in this book. The remainder, I've talked to other people about and have heard success stories for every one of them. These are all methods that you can try to help boost your vagal tone.

Some of these you may already do but need to be more conscious as you do them. Some are new and may require being a bit more open than you have been in the past. For example, if you're not used to acupressure or meditation, these can seem odd and out of place. The great thing about this is that you can pick and choose what you want to try. If one activity isn't the right fit for you, make sure to replace it with something else.

Most people are looking for easy fixes, and while there is no complete cure that doesn't require a little work, you can certainly implement the following methods into your daily life without much effort at all.

Positive Relationships

Your relationships have quite an effect on every aspect of your life, from health and mood to your self-confidence. It's best to surround yourself with positive relationships and people who lift you up. Doing this will not only make you feel happier, but it will also increase your vagus nerve tone and build your immune system.

The vagus nerve is responsible for oxytocin release, the hormone that is essential in human and animal bonding. It makes sense then that it can all affect you when speaking with someone else. If you are talking to someone who is negative or frightens you, then your stress response is activated, your heart rate goes up, and other unpleasant effects occur.

It has also been proven in studies that people who have a higher tone in their vagus nerve tend to be kinder and to bond better with others. If this isn't enough reason to be social, then you might want to look into making more human contact to find out what it feels like. However, this can also be activated when you are around animals. They love unconditionally and can make sure you get lots of positivity.

Regular interaction with other people can lift your spirits an amazing amount. It's easy these days to focus on just being online, but it doesn't count. The technology, while it allows us to communicate, doesn't allow for the person to person interaction that our brains and bodies require.

Getting a genuine hug from someone can tone your vagus nerve. If you get several hugs every day, you'll find that your mood improves. Both eye contact and human touch have massive effects on how toned your vagus nerve is. Every time you spend time with someone else, whether it's laughing over a cup of coffee or holding hands as you walk down the street, your vagus nerve is being stimulated.

Human connection can help you feel calmer, more positive, and improves your mood overall. The effects can last for days, in some situations.

Security and Self-Love

When you feel safe, your vagal tone improves. The same goes for feeling happy and positive. Unfortunately, most people don't really like themselves or their bodies. They find it difficult to take a compliment and will put themselves down. They feel guilty and unhappy about things and are often stressed out, feeling that they just aren't good enough.

Feeling positive about your body and loving who you are can also improve your vagal tone. Self-love is one of the biggest changes you can make in your life, with positive results in your health. You'll find that your immune system functions more efficiently when you are happy with yourself.

Security is another big part of being in control of your life and improving vagal tone. If you feel unsafe, you deal with stress and anxiety. It isn't necessary to have a physical threat right there, though. You can feel stressed if you aren't feeling safe in general. And in today's world, it's very difficult to feel safe. There's always something to worry about.

This was one of the more significant issues that I faced after my vagus nerve was damaged. Before the antibiotic ruined my body, I rarely felt anxious or stressed. All that changed after my vagus nerve was damaged. Suddenly, I was dealing with far more anxiety than before. In addition to the pain, I felt panicky every time I had to do anything outside my comfort zone. Then it got worse. I ended up anxious and stressed over the simplest of things. Even picking my children up from school became a difficult situation. My brain raced over all the things that could go wrong at any given moment and I never truly felt safe.

How can you increase your feeling of security? That depends on the person. In some cases, you may need to take physical steps to make yourself feel safer. This could mean you take the time to install locks on your doors, get a guard dog, etc. These will help you feel safer on the outside. However, you also need to feel secure mentally.

Create a space for yourself where you can relax and detox from the stress of everyday life. This should be an area that reduces anxiety and makes you feel happy and loved. Feeling secure can help your vagus nerve increase tone, so it's worth working on this.

Having a high vagal tone also helps with feeling safe, so it's a cycle that only strengthens as you improve it.

Gratitude

Don't underestimate the power of positive thinking on your vagus nerve health. In fact, it has been proven that a grateful attitude is most prevalent in those with high vagal tone. If your vagal tone is high when you're resting, you are more likely to experience pleasant feelings like gratitude, compassion, love, and will be happier than those with low vagal tone.

You can build on this happiness and increase your vagus nerve tone by developing a habit of being grateful. This is like any other habit, where you need to keep building on it regularly. Here are a few ways you can increase your gratitude:

Keep a gratitude journal: Make a point of writing down at least three things every day that you're grateful for. There will be days when you don't feel like anything is worth saying thanks for, but there is always something. It may be a little thing, like being able to get up in the morning or coffee. There's no shortage of things that you can be thankful for. By focusing on these things every single day, you'll eventually start noticing more things to be grateful for and this will only build.

Say thank you every day: People do things for you every day. Even if they are supposed to do it because it's their job, such as a waitress or bank teller, be sure to say thank you. That little bit of gratitude can have a bit impact, not only on your life, but on other people's lives.

You can even go a bit further if you want, by leaving a generous tip or even a note.

Be with people you love: You can't help but feel grateful and happy when you are around those you love. Make a point of spending time with those special people. Have some tea together, go for a walk, or just sit and chat. You'll find yourself calmer and happier when you spend time with these people.

Be mindful: It's easy to start going through your day on rote, not really thinking about what you're doing as you do the same things you do every day. It's important to stay present as you complete your daily tasks. You can do this by focusing on what you are doing and finding pleasure in the individual task that you are accomplishing. Even doing the dishes can be an enlightening experience if you focus.

Choose happiness: It's important to decide to be happy. This doesn't always work, of course, because you can feel other emotions and sometimes they are more than overwhelming. However, happiness is often a choice and you need to make that choice every day. When you wake up in the morning, take a moment to think about your life and decide that today, you will be happy.

Your daily attitude will have a lot to do with vagal tone. It's also beneficial to your mental attitude to be happy and calm. If it takes raising your vagal tone to do that, then you can start with the exercises I've shared here to get you started.

Diet and Eating Habits

You can improve many aspects of your health simply by eating correctly, but did you know that this also has a massive effect on your vagus nerve? I didn't realize until after I had already changed my eating habits that there were some other benefits to this lifestyle, including boosting vagal tone.

It turns out that what you eat and the bacteria in your digestive tract actually affect how your brain functions. The bacteria in your gut can get upset or become imbalanced when you take antibiotics or other types of medicines. That's exactly what happened to me. So when my friend told me to take probiotics, she was actually on the right track. It just takes more than a few bottles of kombucha to fix the gut.

What Foods Should You Eat?

The types of foods you eat are very important, but some are more so. Here are some foods that should be included in your daily diet:

Fermented Food: Fermented foods include healthy microbes and bacteria, so they can help restore your digestive tract bacteria if it has been depleted. Things like sauerkraut, cheese, kefir, kombucha, and yogurt are some of the more common fermented foods. However, you can also make fermented salsa, ketchup, and many other delicious, gut-boosting foods at home.

Foods High in Fiber: You want to keep things moving and one of the signs that your gut is not healthy is constipation. It makes sense then to eat fiber, but there's another good reason for this . . . prebiotics. Your high fiber foods contain prebiotics that will help good gut bacteria flourish and reduce your stress levels. High fiber foods include anything made with whole grains, seeds, fruits and vegetables, and nuts.

Calcium: Known as the bone-building mineral, calcium helps protect the body against diseases like diabetes and cancer. It's also an essential part of keeping your nervous system and cardiovascular system functioning properly, which includes your vagus nerve. Calcium is one of the nutrients that the body cannot produce, so you need to eat it. You'll find calcium in dairy products, dark green leafy vegetables like kale or broccoli, and in canned fish with softened bones.

Magnesium: Without magnesium, the heart cannot function as well as it should. In fact, this mineral is an essential part of regulating the circulatory system. It helps the heart contract correctly, manages heart rhythm and prevents many cardiac issues. It can be found in nuts and seeds, green leafy vegetables like kale and spinach, figs, avocado, bananas, and seafood in general. Legumes such as beans and peas are also rich in magnesium.

Sodium: Chances are you've heard that salt is bad for you all your life. It's a common misconception and, while too much sodium isn't great for the body, it is necessary for your body to function. Whole grain bread, cured meats, and chicken are all excellent sources of sodium. You can also use sea salt or Himalayan salt in your food.

Why Is Important To Organise A Good Routine And Don't Ignore Hobbies And Passions

Finally, let's talk practical exercises that'll change your vagus nerve's state. Exercising is very important for the body, but did you know it could stimulate the vagus nerve too/ here, we'll discuss practical exercises that'll stimulate your vagus nerve, and some of the different aspects that go along with this type of nerve.

Yoga

First, let's talk about yoga. Yoga is one of the simplest exercises to stimulate the vagus nerve, but not only that, it's wonderful for promoting bodily relaxation and general wellness.

Yoga requires you to do small positions, whether it be downward dog, different hand and foot positions, or even a simple lotus position. What you do while doing this, is focus on your breathing. You're encouraged to have even, soft breathing from your diaphragm, and also to hold the position, feeling your muscles at first tense, but then relax as you hold it for longer.

Yoga is one of the single best ways to stimulate your vagus nerve. It's simple, it doesn't take much, to begin with it, and you don't have to do it for a long period of time. It is a form of exercise, and it's calming.

But, don't underestimate yoga. It can be quite powerful. Some people struggle with it, simply because it's oftentimes long, and you might not be used to these various positions. It's quite freeing though, and it liberates you.

If you're someone who only has a little bit of time for physical activity every day, then try yoga. There are many variants to it too, many positions that'll stimulate your vagus nerve just by doing them and holding them, and that's something that most don't realize.

The Power of Yoga Nidra

One aspect of yoga that's worth mentioning is yoga Nidra. This is one of the best types of yoga practices since it lets you naturally restore your body, along with your mind via unlocking and touching upon your parasympathetic nervous system. It is a slow practice, but incredibly powerful, and very helpful for building better wellness, and understanding of your vagus nerve.

How do you do it through? Well first, you want to get int a comfortable position, whether with a blanket or a mat. From there close your eyes, and start to breathe. Start to become aware of your breathing, and space and the feelings you possess. From there, sit there, and hold that position, focusing on the breathing.

You can lay down, you can have your legs crossed, you can have them sit up. Literally, just sit down, and from there, relax. This is nourishing, this is filling, and it's a relaxing experience too.

Hold the position for as long as you want, but usually, about 30 minutes is more than enough.

The Power of Stretching

Let's talk about stretching. This doe tie into yoga, but if you combine diaphragmic breathing with yoga. Doing this as you do a mall stretch, it'll benefit you in a ton of different ways. For starters, most people don't stretch nearly enough, and it shows. Most people aren't flexible, and it affects how they end up faring in life. Many get injured due to a lack of stretching.

But, it's more than that. stretching is powerful. Stretching is used in order to help naturally stimulate the body, and make movement simple. There is a lot that you can achieve from this, and a lot that you can get out of this. Most people don't realize that when they stretch, they're not only releasing tensions within the muscles, but they're also focusing their breathing so that it's simple, and yet very effective.

A lot of people don't stretch enough, so that tension sits there. But, a way to naturally start up the parasympathetic nervous system and activate et vagus nerve is to do just this. Sitting down, stretching out your body, and working on this helps promote relaxation and wellness, and from there will stimulate your entire body in its own way.

Plus, it feels amazing too. Most people don't stretch enough, and they'll realize as they do this, that they really need to. Sometimes having calming music, and focusing on your breathing changes this.

You also don't have to hold the stretches for very long. About 10-12 seconds suffices.

Try touching your toes, stretching your arms behind your head, pushing them up and holding your arms in the air, or even just moving towards your foot will help with this. There is a lot of benefits to be had with stretching, and a lot of wonderful things to do with this. You'll be shocked, you'll be amazed, and most of all, you'll be quite happy with the power of this small exercise, and you'll feel invigorated for whatever is to come next for you in the future.

Consider stretching right before you begin your day, or at the end of the night, and see how it helps you feel during the day, and you'll feel your vagus nerve stimulate almost immediately.

Weight Training

Weight training might seem weird to do in order to stimulate the vagus nerve, but it does work. That's because, when you lift weights, it is changing the speed of the body. Plus, through the power of repetition, you get your body to relax. A lot of people think lifting weights is only for big, burly people, but that isn't the case.

Ever just doing a few sets of curls will change the way your body feels, and your vagus nerve. So many people also think they need to start off with a heavy weight right away but that isn't the case. I suggest just progressively overloading over time if you want to see physical gains, but understand that weight training is a relaxing process, and you breathe as you do it. You need to breathe in deeply in order to help with pushing the oxygen around to help you with strenuous exercise. So yes, pick up that dumbbell, and try it. You'll feel the difference right away.

HIIT Workouts

HIIT, or "high intensity interval training" is a form of workouts that require you to do a lot in a very small period of time. Sometimes, this involves sprinting, other times this can be pushups, situps, or other exercises. The main goal behind this is to do a lot in a little bit of time, and through spurts.

These sprits are what cause vagus nerve stimulation. The vagus nerve is usually not stimulated if you're constantly stressed out, but the periods of stress, and then relaxation will kick the vagus nerve into gear, helping it activate whenever it's needed.

HIIT workouts are also great because they are oftentimes very easy to do. No matter what it is that you do, you'll feel the difference in these immediately.

A lot of people don't realize that HIIT is also very short in terms of workouts. Some people can get these done within a half hour or so, and that's their workout for the day. But HIIT is great because it lets you get a great workout, but also lets you improve your own personal wellness, and health too.

It's a great way to get in shape, so it's something you should consider if you're looking to improve your physical fitness.

Walking

Walking is a great option if you're not into going to the gym to lift, or you don't want to spend time doing HIIT or yoga. Walking is a good habit to get into because it stimulates your body and helps with physical fitness and wellness. Your vagus nerve will get stimulated with walking, especially if you live a sedentary lifestyle.

I think walking for 30 minutes a day is ideal, especially if you're unable to do this otherwise. Sometimes, walking while on your breaks is a great way to do this, and walking also lets you improve on your own personal health and wellness. You want to do this to help with your physical fitness, and walking is a good start, especially if you're not active otherwise.

Jogging is also another good one because this can help with deep breathing. A lot of people, when they start, will get into the habit of breathing with short breaths, but that won't work here. This can actually make it hard to run, and you might pass out. With jogging, you want to make sure that you're breathing in a slow, deep, and even manner, and focus on this. This will help with your vagus nerve, and also help you get into the habit of breathing deeply. You can also do running with this, but it's more high-intensity and might be harder to engage in deep breathing otherwise.

Jumping

Again, another form of cardio that's great, but, your vagus nerve will love it. Jumping jacks, burpees, and other jumping exercises are good because it will help with improving circulation, which can help with blood pressure and your vagal tone.

When you jump too, be mindful of your breathing. Try to do it with deep breathing, and you'll notice it's a much harder workout, but you'll feel the difference. It also increases blood flow, blood pressure, and heart rate as well.

Your vagus nerve will thank you for this, and you'll be able to, with jumping too, improve on your own personal health and wellness too.

Aerobics

Aerobics is another higher-intensity exercise, but there are variants that aren't as extensive and as intensive as others. Zumba tends to be on the more intensive side, but there are different classes you can try. However, there are even different kinds of aerobics exercises you can do, such as water aerobics, weight training, cycling, and even yoga. All of these when combined, are wonderful for vagus nerve stimulation and are great for the body. You'll be amazed and surprised at how helpful this can be for the body, and how you can use these to help improve your vagus nerve. They encourage you to breathe during these too, which encourages deep breathing, and thereby vagus nerve stimulation.

Swim it Out!

Swimming is a great aerobic exercise too, and if you're not a fan of jogging or running, or weight training, swimming is good.

That's because it actually helps in many different ways. For starters, you're submerging your head, which stimulates the mammalian diving reflex, which includes your vagus nerve. It also pushes you to control your breathing as you move. You need to hold your breath, but also move through the water, and it's a combination of both of those things which provides you with the correct vagus nerve stimulation.

It also will help improve your bodily movement. That's because, you're moving about, and this encourages blood flow too. You'll notice that as you begin with this, at first, it's hard to do, but over time, you'll get better with this. It's a wonderful form of cardio, and it's wonderful for properly stimulating the vagus nerve.

Dancing

Finally, we have dancing. Dancing is a great form of self-expression for starters, and even if you're being silly, it can help you feel much better about yourself. Dance is wonderful because it helps you improve your physical fitness, get the blood flow moving, and help you stay active and fun.

There are so many different kinds of dance classes these days too. You can do Zumba or other forms of dancing. Some people even like ballet dancing because it requires control, and this can stimulate the vagus nerve. They're fun to do, and they encourage you to move, control your breathing, and also let you express yourself.

Even silly interpretive dancing helps. After all, if it can make you laugh, that naturally stimulates the vagus nerve, and that's a wonderful, fun way to do this. Dancing is great, and it lets you feel good about yourself. Definitely consider dancing next time you want to properly express yourself, and feel good.

When it comes to stimulating the vagus nerve, these are all practice activities to help with stimulating the vagus nerve. Your vagus nerve is very important because it lets you relax the body, and helps curb inflammation. But, while these exercises are great for stimulating this, it also helps with getting the body moving, which increases vagal tone. It can also help offset obesity, diabetes, and other conditions related to weight.

Your vagus nerve does benefit from exercise, and here, we discussed why and how it happens, and the benefits of this.

Few Tips To Have A Good Routine

The following exercises will help tone your vagus nerve for long-term efficiency. These exercises should be incorporated daily or at least weekly into your regular routine. Many are simple exercises or activities that can be done in a few minutes; others focus on making lifestyle changes that will strengthen the vagus nerve.

Body Awareness

Be more aware of your thoughts, the sensation of your body, and your emotional experiences. Ways to increase body awareness can be accomplished through:

- Tai chi
- Yoga
- Emotional journaling
- Body breathing exercises
- Thought journaling.

Body scanning meditation is a highly effective way to be more aware of your body and can also be used to reduce stress and eliminate tension in the body. It also strengthens the mind-body connection. To perform a body scan meditation, something you want to take note of are the sensations you might feel such as:

- Tingling
- Itching
- Pain
- Pulsing
- Cold spots
- Hot spots
- Tightness
- Cramping
- Nausea
- Numbness.

You want to dedicate at least 30 minutes to this exercise once or twice a week. To perform a body scan exercise:

1. Begin in a lying position with the eyes closed or at least half-closed.

2. Bring your focus to your breath. Take note of how the air fills your body and the way your body feels as you

exhale. In what areas do you feel pressure? Where do you feel relaxed?

3.   After focusing on your breathing, you want to move your attention down to your toes. Take notice of any sensations you might feel as you focus on each individual toe. When you come across any sensation, stop and take note. If any muscles or areas feel tense, take your time to let them relax.

4.   From the toes move to the balls of your feet. Is there pain or tingling?

5.   Then move across the bottom of the feet to the heels. Again stop and take note of what sensations you may feel.

6.   Then move across to the tops of your feet and then to the ankles. Do you feel pain or swelling? Or do they feel relaxed and limber?

7.   Make your way up the calves, focusing on the muscles as you go. Do they feel tense?

8.   Next focus on the knees.

9.   Continue to scan across the entirety of your body until you reach the crown of your head. Once you have covered all areas, muscles, and vital organs, take a few

more deep breaths in and out. Your body should be relaxed and you mind should feel clear.

If at any point during this process you notice your focus has shifted elsewhere, simple guide it back to where you left off. It can be challenging to maintain focus for the entirety of this meditation but the more you practice, the longer you will be able to maintain your focus where it is supposed to be and the easier it will be to bring it back.

Environmental Awareness

Bringing awareness to your environment will help you identify your environment as a safe space. One of the best ways to bring more awareness to your environment is through mindfulness meditation. This can be done while sitting in your environment or while walking through it. Clear your thoughts and tune into your sense. Begin by putting your focus on what you hear. Since the vagus nerve links up to the inner ear, you are causing it to activate from the start of the process when you put your attention on what you are hearing. Take note of all the sounds you hear; what animals do you hear? What noise do you hear when the wind blows? Are their children playing nearby?

Once you go through the sounds you pick up, move to your sense of smell; again take a mental note of what you smell. How do the smells make you feel? If you catch yourself thinking negative thoughts or your focus shifting to thoughts and are not dealing with the environment you are in currently, simply let the thoughts go and bring your focus back to the present moment. Continue this process until you have gone through each of the senses.

Diet

Figure 25: Free Image

Eating a balanced, healthy diet keeps your whole system in check, but is even more important for keeping your digestive tract working properly. A diet that is whole food and plant-based eliminates toxins, chemicals, and unhealthy ingredients that can cause inflammation in the digestive tract and throw off hormone production. Your diet should consist of:

- Organic vegetables, especially dark leafy greens, as they are rich in fiber and aid digestion.

- Fresh fruits; berries are ideal, as they have the least amount of natural sugars compared to other fruits.

Apples are also a healthy choice as they are rich in fiber, which slows down the absorption of the sugar it contains.

- Omega-3 rich fish, like salmon, sardines, and tuna, are great sources of protein and omega-3 fatty acids, which promote brain health.

- Nuts and seeds are great snacks and contain healthy fats and proteins.

- Whole grains, like quinoa, barley, and steel cuts oats, provide fiber and additional nutrients to the body that help regulate digestion and promote overall gut health.

Your diet should reduce or eliminate:

- Alcohol

- Spicy food

- Processed food

- Trans fats

- Additives

- Prepacked foods

- Sugar

- White flour products such as bread, rice, and cereals.

These items can cause irritation to the digestive tract and result in irritation of the vagus nerve.

Probiotics

Probiotics are needed to help heal the gut and maintain healthy gut bacteria. This can reduce inflammation of the digestive tract that can cause irritation of the vagus nerve. They promote healthy gut bacteria growth to better allow the vagus nerve to produce the feel-good hormones and neurotransmitters that will keep you in a rest and digest response. Probiotics can be consumed in a supplement form or by including fermented foods into your diet such as:

- Kombucha, fermented tea

- Kifer, a cultured milk with added kefir grains. It is similar to yogurt

- Tempeh, fermented soybean

- Kimchi, fermented cabbage, radish, or other vegetables

- Sauerkraut, fermented cabbage

- Yogurt, fermented milk.

Daily Activities

Exercise is essential for maintaining healthy vagus nerve stimulation. Include a variety of exercise routines that can keep you in optimal shape and keep your vagus nerve properly stimulated. Exercises can range from low impact to high intensity. The goal is to get about 30 minutes of movement, three to five days a week. Yoga, tai chi, and aerobics should be a part of your exercise schedule. These not only help keep the parasympathetic system active but also helps train the vagus nerve to regulate proper breathing and heart rate control.

Physical activities are not the only way you can include exercise into your day. While physical activity is vital for overall health, including brain-stimulating activities or movement controlled/coordination activities are also beneficial. These types of activities can help strengthen the connection between the vagus nerve and the brain, making it easier for signals to pass to and from the nerve, brain, and the rest of the body.

Yoga

Yoga stimulates the vagus nerve through deep breathing exercises and focused movements. Yoga can have a powerful impact on reducing symptoms of depression, anxiety, and chronic pain. Making yoga a regular part of your daily routine can also lead to a reduction of stress, better sleep, and improved digestion. Yoga can also be beneficial for those with autism spectrum disorder, ADHD, or sensory processing disorder because it strengthens your body awareness.

One of the best yoga moves for vagal toning is the cat-cow pose. This pose stretches the spin, allowing it to come into proper alignment while stimulating the digestive tract. To perform this pose:

1. Begin in a tabletop position on the floor on the knees and hands. The wrist should align below the shoulders and the knees should align below the hips, hip-width apart. The fingers should be pointed toward the front. Bring your head to a center neutral position with your gaze toward the ground just slightly in front of you.

2. Take a deep breath in as you lower your abdomen towards the floor and lift the chest and chin up. Shift

your gaze from the floor to the ceiling. Allow the shoulders to widen, pulling them away from the ears.

3. Exhale as you bring the abdomen back up and round the spine as if you were a cat stretching your back. Lower your head back down to the floor but not entirely; you want to avoid bringing the chin to the chest.

4. On the inhale, repeat the second step. On the exhale, repeat the third step.

5. Do this process five times. When finished, bring yourself to a seated position, resting on the heels and lifting the torso slowly up. Take a few deep inhales and exhales before standing.

Improve Your Posture

Poor posture can lead to a weaker vagus nerve. It can put you at greater risk of developing hiatal hernias, hinder the digestive system, and place unnecessary stress and strain on the neck. This makes it more difficult for signals to be sent to and from the vagus nerve to be transmitted properly. Tips for improving your posture include:

- Stand straight and tall with your body weight primarily in the balls of your feet. Keep the feet about hip-width apart and be sure to tuck in the butt and stomach.

- Refrain from slouching or slumping.

- Avoid looking down at your phone for long periods of time.

- Wear comfortable shoes that support the arch and cushion the heel and balls of your feet.

Breathing Exercises

Learning to regulate your breathing is one of the most effective ways to tone the vagus nerve. Stimulating the vagus nerve can be immediately done by taking a few deep breaths. This can be used as an effective way to reduce stress, counter anxiety, and reduce inflammation. When you inhale deeply, your trigger the relaxation response in the body, but it is the exhaling that allows for the vagus nerve to become activated. When you are able to control and slow down the exhale, you will strengthen vagal tone and be able to more quickly utilize its power.

Proper breathing when your vagus nerve is in optimal condition is accomplished when you take a breath in and out six times a minute. This is done by inhaling and exhaling for the same length of time, five seconds for each. This is the goal when toning the vagus nerve but the focus should primarily rely on slowing the breath, feeling calm, and bringing balance to the mind and body. When you focus on slowing the breath, it will, in most instances, naturally fall into a six breaths per minute pattern.

In order to achieve this proper breathing pattern, you can begin by toning the vagus nerve through a simple deep breathing technique. Begin by inhaling a long and slow breaths for seven seconds each. As you inhale, focus on allowing the air to fill your belly or abdomen. Once you have inhaled deeply, hold the breath for a second or two, and then slowly exhale for 10 seconds. The inhaling and exhaling should be done through the nose. You should repeat this process six times until you can properly breathe in and out for up to 12 times.

Healthy Connections

Hugging has been shown to stimulate the vagus nerve. Making regular healthy connections, and having meaningful and fulfilling relationships, can help tone the vagus nerve on a regular basis. Maintaining a healthy connection can be as simple as sending a few friendly text messages to having a long in-depth conversation with a close advisor or friend. When you initiate conversation, you're creating a balance between the sympathetic nervous system and parasympathetic system and mastering the process of transitioning from freeze and/or fight or flight to social engagement phases.

Conclusion

The vagus nerve assumes a fundamental job in our general wellbeing and prosperity. As a business person, you've presumably felt the impacts of the physiological reactions it administers without acknowledging it – especially during distressing periods.

"Hacking" your vagus nerve is extremely about embracing a couple of solid practices that keep it invigorated and working ideally. There are more procedures we could plunge into, yet those recorded are probably the most straightforward to actualize and have strong logical support. You can take full breaths from your office!

The vagus nerve is one, if not, the most important neural network in the human body. It controls a number of systems which are vital to the overall functioning of the body's essential biological functions. That means that if the vagus nerve does not perform up to its optimal capabilities, the effects on the overall functioning of the body can be significant. Hence, there is a great need for everyone to understand how it works, what it does and what can be done to ensure that it functions up to its full potential.

Moreover, the vagus nerve is not fully understood. Its incredible power hasn't been fully understood until recently. Modern research has revealed the importance of this nerve and the need for its care. This has given way to a score of approaches with the aim to keep the vagus nerve in peak performance. In this book, we will discuss these approaches as a means of ensuring that we are able to maintain optimal health and wellbeing, both of the vagus nerve itself, and by extension, the body systems that it controls.

This book has been written with the intent to inform the general public on this topic. So, even a novice in the topic of the nervous system will be able to make the most of this important issue. After all, we are not here to provide complex information; rather, our intent is to provide you with information you won't easily find anywhere else.

As such, this book has been written with the aim of allowing anyone who is interested in learning about the topic the opportunity to do so in plain language. This book isn't an attempt at trying to sound smart; it is an exercise in helping the average individual learn as much as they can in a clear and concise manner. That means that we are going to be getting down to the meat and potatoes of this topic straight from the get-go.

This is an important consideration especially since the vagus nerve is indeed the body's main control module. Also, given the fact that we tend to know very little about it, we end up ignoring its relevance in our overall health and wellbeing. When we understand what this nerve does in our body, we are able to make a conscious choice to ensure its health. In doing so, we can keep a good level of physical wellbeing.

If you do happen to experience the ill effects of one of the more ceaseless incendiary conditions, vagus nerve incitement through electrical driving forces shows a ton of guarantee. This might be something to explore and raise with your medical expert.

www.ingramcontent.com/pod-product-compliance
Lightning Source LLC
Chambersburg PA
CBHW071405210526
45465CB00001B/263